Mental

A Student Nurse Account

Jack Bennington

chipmunkapublishing

the mental health publisher

Published by

Chipmunkapublishing

PO Box 6872

Brentwood

Essex CM13 1ZT

United Kingdom

http://www.chipmunkapublishing.com

Chipmunkapublishing gratefully acknowledge the support of Arts Council England.

For Helen,

who gave me the strength and confidence to

carry on when times were tough.

And to Mike, for the inspired chats.

Jack Bennington

Author Biography

Jack Bennington was born in 1977 in the West Midlands. He gained a degree in Film, T.V, and Radio Studies in early 2000 but, after developing an interest in psychology, later trained as a Mental Health Nurse in 2007. Upon qualifying in 2010 he took up a position working with individuals with Dementia. Jack continues to develop his interest and knowledge of mental health issues, in particular the link between healthy living and psychology. He still works closely with his local university in developing educational and visual training tools for future mental health students.

Jack Bennington

Times are often tough in mental health, and there are days where you do question your ability to go on, or even your own well being, doing a job like this day in and day out. But equally, as with most jobs, you find a hidden inner strength to carry on, and find that some days you really have felt that you have made a difference in someone's life, be that just affording someone five or ten minutes to sit down with them and talk about their life and experiences. It is in those rare snapshots and time frames that you begin to uncover the 'real' person behind the illness. Working within dementia is not easy, and not for the faint hearted, but if we can be there for someone in their time of need, the rewards are often magical in their nature, providing a warm glow inside us, which in turn helps our own well being. There have been laughs, and there have been tears. I hope you enjoy reading this book, and appreciate the range of experiences and insight that I have been lucky to experience throughout my training. Whilst it is easy to quickly become quite cynical, particularly within the 'daily grind' of the ward environment, let us not forget that when we can go home at the end of a long and hard shift, many of our patients can no longer afford such a luxury, and for them, they are home. Let us embrace our skills and experience and step back and remember who we are really there for.

All of the following is true. Names have been changed to protect confidentiality. Anecdotes and situations were all lived through my own eyes. This is real life, and what it's truly like to be a student mental health nurse.

This account is in no way making fun of or demeaning the staff or patients within the mental health system. It is merely intended as a factual account of a student nurse's journey through training and some of the thought processes during this time period. It is in no way making fun of mental illness.

At the time of writing the training for a RMN is three years in duration, with 3 placements in a variety of areas each year to expose you to the wide spectrum of experiences within mental health.

Enjoy the journey.

Jack Bennington

Jack Bennington

Jack Bennington

7am – 9am

As I look at my alarm clock, which is blaring away at me with a horrible robotic sound, I realised I had pushed the snooze button about 3 times already and now it was reading 7.10am. I had to be in work in 35 minutes. It took me at least 15 minutes to drive over to the hospital, which meant I only had about 20 minutes to get changed, do all the normal bathroom chores and try to gulp a cup of coffee and grab some toast.

This was my final placement area of a three year mental health nurse training course. Many of my colleagues had felt like quitting during various parts of the course. In fact some had. It certainly wasn't for everyone, and at times I had found my will to carry on with the course had waned at various junctures, but thanks to a combination of supportive colleagues and lecturers, I had battled through. I now had this final placement area left. An elderly dementia ward, which at full capacity contained fourteen patients. I had sensed the feeling of dread the night before, because I knew it was the other team working today's shift. The ward had two teams working a day shift, and two teams working a night shift. This would normally consist of at least two qualified mental health nurses and three nursing assistants, and possibly additional agency staff. These agency staff had been getting a bad name lately. A lot of the time they seemed to be booked randomly to a ward they had never worked on before, which meant the nurses and nursing assistants had a harder time as they had to explain the basic running of the ward and the patients to them before they had started. A lot of the time I had heard them being described as 'as useful as a plank of wood'. A lot of the nurses would bad mouth them behind their back. I had decided to not get into this political minefield and just keep my head down and get on with things. I had no real complaints about them myself, except for maybe one day when I was trying to get on with my work, but one of the staff known only as 'NT' wanted to discuss the finer details of internet role play gaming and how he had spent most of his previous weeks staying up all night playing some war wizard and amassing lots of hit points.

I had got lucky so far in being with the better of the two teams, but I knew that Linda was on today. I just couldn't stand the woman. She had already made my life hell by pestering me for the whole duration of a twelve hour shift, and it had worn me down. I had heard horror stories in the past of her reducing first year students to tears. I had previously worked with her the week before, and it was a nightmare. I didn't sit down for a second, and was continually being barked at like an army cadet.

I drag myself out of bed and quickly change into my well worn white polo shirt, the industry standard. I didn't care for it much, but the tunics I detested even more. In fact I still had three pristine packaged tunics tucked away in the corner of my wardrobe, along with the truly awful school grey trousers, which I had worn a few times, but they were just too long, and as a man, I've had to claim a huge failure by not knowing how to 'turn up' such items. The tunics had remained packaged, as they just looked like my own version of a straightjacket. I detested uniforms enough as it was, but I was loathe to try on something that looked like it had been made with one hundred percent pure starch.

My name badge was still intact, clearly labelling me as the 'student nurse', a badge I would be unable to hide behind for too much longer as I was nearing the end of the placements. I put on my black Nike trainers, a cunning new plan to get out of wearing proper shoes. I had tried shoes for a few twelve hour shifts, and my feet had just come back sweating and aching. This way my new shiny Nike trainers would not arouse suspicion and would cleverly blend in to look like real shoes. I figure if I'm going to do twelve hour shifts, it might as well be in comfort.

I glance at the clock on the DVD player in my living room; 7.22am. I'm not going to have time for a cup of coffee. Why do I never get up in time? Instead I continually rush round the house, stuffing cheap wholemeal toast into my mouth whilst developing a sweat induced anxiety state. I have only myself to blame, but I just never start the morning on a very good footing.

Still feeling the sense of dread of the shift ahead of me, I walk out of the house and sit in my car, and decide on the next few tunes on my iPod that will try to lift my mood for the short journey from my house to the hospital. I was in quite an angry mood lately, so the last few journeys I had been listening to a lot of Rage Against The Machine, a suitably good album to fire you up, but maybe not the best thing to play at the start of the shift; it probably wouldn't get me in the right sort of mood. Instead I opt for a much calmer choice, and go with some Coldplay.

It was winter, another reason why I had trouble getting out of bed for a long shift ahead of me. As I drive towards my destination for the next twelve hours, I notice a man walking his dog, a mother taking her two daughters to school, a squirrel darting around the bottom of a large oak tree, the leaves glistening with last night's rainfall. I wished that I was doing anything but going to work. I had been having these feelings for some time now; it was not the easiest placement that I had been assigned to, it was elderly care, working with a variety of patients with similar brain degeneration such as Alzheimer's, and dementia. A difficult ward, and not the area I was particularly wanting to move towards as a career, but I had to be placed on this ward as you need a wide variety of experiences within your training, so there was no choice in the matter. I was suffering through it, the placement was twelve weeks in total, and this was my ninth week. These mornings of dread and anxiety were becoming far too frequent.

I arrived at the hospital, by which time I had managed about three and a half songs from Coldplay, which I wasn't sure had entirely fixed my mood, but it had given me a suitable distraction for the duration of the trip. I hadn't really been focussing on where I was driving to, my feet just knew when to push the pedals, and my arms automatically manoeuvred the steering wheel. I was on autopilot. The car park was deserted; only a few other cars were parked up at this early hour.

The hospital was a listed building and it had been here for a good 200 years. In the old days it was a lunatic asylum. I dread to think of the things that went on back in those days. Back in the 1960s there had been a terrible fire on one of the wards, which had wiped out an entire ward of patients. This had sparked the well worn rumour that the place was haunted, something that I just couldn't bring myself to believe in until I had concrete proof on the matter. Many times a nursing assistant would tell me that they saw an 'actual' ghost floating past them, or curious mist emanating from the bottom of a patient's door. As a complete sceptic I just couldn't bring myself to believe the stories; just because so many people kept telling me about them didn't mean they were true. It was bitterly cold in the car park, and the sky was still a murky grey colour. It was a short walk through to the ward and I would often see one of the ward managers standing by his large black Range Rover, having a cigarette as I made my way to the ward. He always dressed in a sharp black suit, and wore small round spectacles, with an inch thick goatee beard surrounding the middle of his face. I had met him briefly on another placement area, but he didn't like students, rarely even giving them eye contact. Today was no exception as I walked past him, and carried on to the ward.

I take a big deep breath, and put the key in the first large green door, and lock it behind me. I open the inner door, which opens directly onto the ward, and step into the corridor. The bright white lights immediately hit me, and the familiar smell of lightly fragranced cleaning products. On the wall nearest to the entrance were pictures of all the nursing team, and their names, all encased in a large glass frame. It reminded me of old school photographs you had to have each year. Each picture was the member of staff's face, complete with awkward smile. There were still many empty spaces within the frame, and not all the staff members pictures were actually in this, almost a half hearted attempt to look professional. Staff members changed so much these days and were regularly moved onto other wards.

I look right in front of me; the office door is slightly ajar, I can see lots of movement from behind the white frosted glass door. I always hated walking into the office, I'm not really sure why, maybe it's the fact that I always seem to be the last in there. The office is small and cramped and all the staff are in there having a drink already. It feels awkward as you have to sort of hunch yourself up and stand around whilst the night staff hand over any important information about the patients during the night. The office is a mess; there are bits of paper strewn all over the desk. I am standing in front of the big whiteboard which details all the current patients that are on the ward and any special requirements, for example if they are diabetic, or allergic to anything, and if they are on a soft/pureed diet, as they might be at risk of choking. It also details if they are for resuscitation, if they are not then it clearly states 'DNR', and in a bright shade of red, this means that we as staff are not to try and aid in their resuscitation and let them die as comfortably as possible.

The night staff always look considerably weary. I don't blame them, they have in effect completely reversed their circadian rhythm which isn't really a natural thing to do at all; the bleary eyes say it all. Susan, the night nurse, is detailing any important information about the patients, Susan is an 'old school nurse'. Coming straight from school at 16, she has worked here for the past 33 years, and is well grounded in her routine, she seeks no further ambition now and is just waiting till her retirement day, which won't be happening for a further six years. There is nothing much to tell today. Everyone has slept well throughout the night, and only a few have got up to go to the toilet. She hands over the keys to the day nurse, Linda. There is only Linda in charge today, the other nurse rang in sick late last night, and there has been no one available to cover the shift. Linda gives me a look up and down, as if she is analysing every microbe of my clothing. She tries to smile, but her zygomatic major muscles are not being activated, meaning there are no creases in the corner of her eyes, hence she is delivering to me her best fake smile. Linda has deep blue eyes, and a small brown bob of hair, which is neatly parted down the middle to exacting precision. In her mid 40's, she has some slight signs of ageing around the eyes, but generally the years have been kind to her.

Andrew is here at least. Andrew is a nursing assistant, originally from Spain, and he is a remarkable character, with short jet black hair, the trademark Tom Cruise style grin, and his use of the word 'lovely'. He never shows signs of faltering and he will often do four long shifts in a row, dealing with everything that is thrown at him. I have never seen him get angry or stressed, and all the patients seem to like him. I liked being on shift with Andrew. When you were feeling down, you really appreciated that smile, and he would always have a handful of jokes on tap to provide you with some amusement during the day. He fancied himself as a bit of a ladies' man too, he would often flirt with most of the female staff, particularly the nursing assistants or agency staff, and would usually have all sorts of tales from his past about his various sexual adventures that he used to get up to, which again would really help the day fly by.

And at least he cared more for students than Linda. 'Hey', he beckons to me, 'Make yourself a drink, why don't you'. 'Sure' I say, it was nice to actually be asked. Linda looked in disgust at the very mention of someone being a little civil to students. The diary is opened by Linda. The daily diary will detail any important events or tasks that need to be done throughout the day, which can mean a whole manner of things including taking patients to x-ray, or ringing up the pharmacy to arrange leave medications for patients that have been granted some time off the ward (this rarely happens with the end stages of dementia sadly), and if there are any other medical interventions required whilst on the ward, and any doctors that need contacting. The daily diary was the first point of contact for every shift.

Linda scours the diary, and starts speaking to me. 'Malcolm will need his leave meds arranged, you can ring pharmacy for that as you're a third year student can't you, you can also ring the doctor and arrange for Cybil to be looked at, her feet are swollen, I'll keep you busy today don't you worry'.

What I truly detested about Linda was the *way* in which she spoke to me. Linda wasn't exactly an old school nurse, in fact she was fairly new out of the box so to speak and had only been qualified two years, which is why I had no idea why she used to speak to me in this way and boss me about. Just the tone of her voice seemed to garner some outright glee in telling me what I could do for her, and that she was able to keep me busy for the duration of the day. I smiled and simply said 'Sure'. I wasn't going to let her grind me down like she had other students. The best policy I figured was to just do everything I was asked, keep my head down and finish the placement without incident. I wasn't going to let her think she could beat me or gradually wear me down, I wasn't going to break, I had gone through enough to get this far, and this was the final hurdle, my last placement before qualifying and she was not going to get in my way. You seemed to find as a student that nurses could go either way. You would get the nurses who had equally had a bad time during their training and would like to pass on their misery or hardship to you, because that's just the 'way things were' for them. Then you would get the other more helpful sort that realised that nurse training could really be a real struggle at times, and you really needed support and just someone to talk to and offer help and advice. Linda was not one of those nurses. Whatever experiences she had as a student certainly couldn't have been pleasant as she seemed to have great delight in passing on whatever misery she had experienced over to me.

After we had drunk our tea it was time to go and get the patients up. Linda was going to work with Andrew, and Linda had quite abruptly told me I was going to work with one of the agency girls who had just turned up. She was a very small Japanese girl, whom I had seen before on the ward. Her name was Valencia, and she was incredibly timid and hardly uttered a word. I was pleased to not be working with Linda anyway, she never chose to work with me and that suited me just fine. There would often be agency staff on the ward, despite a fully rostered staff rota. Sickness was a particular problem within the trust, and most notably in the winter time. I would often have to get used to working with a lot of different people whilst on shift with varying skills and experience. 'You go and get Malcolm up this morning, and the rest of the men, OK Luvee', Linda ordered at me. Why did she have the need to add 'luvee' at the end of the sentence I have no idea, but I grit my teeth and walk out with Valencia. I ask 'Have you worked on this ward before?'

'Yes' she utters in a very childlike manner. I look at the clock. It was 8.10am, the day was only just beginning and already I just felt like going home and crawling up in a ball playing Xbox all day long. I tried to snap myself out of this feeling, and concentrate on the day ahead.

The sluice room. Before entering the sluice room we have to go to a room which contains small silver bowls on wheels, two tiered. The lower bowl was so that you could stack it full of your morning requirements for each patient. Usually a cardboard urine bottle, some wipes, and a pad (which resemble a large adult nappy). The top bowl was for warm water. I take a bowl and wheel it unconvincingly into the sluice room, where we have to put on a plastic apron and some gloves. Andrew is trying to chat up the agency worker again. 'Hey lovely, you working here all day long ?' Valencia smiles and again says a simple 'yes' in the quietest voice ever. Andrew is married but he likes to flirt with the staff, it gets him through the day, and the staff don't seem to mind it. Andrew turns to me and hands me a plastic apron. 'And how you doing today Mr?'. 'Oh just fine' I lie unconvincingly. 'Just a bit tired really, that's all'. 'Ah, you been having a late night again sir ?' Andrew asks. 'Nah, not really, just all these shifts catching up with me that's all'. 'Don't worry, you have the weekend off anyway don't you ?' Andrew grins. 'Yeh, I sure do, can't wait'. Andrew smiles, as he wheels out his bowl of fresh hot water and goes into one of the patient's rooms. Linda walks past me not looking me in the eye. She stops just in the doorway, and turns to me. 'Oh, you can do some more care plans for me today and some risk assessments can't you ?' 'Yes, no problem' I said. She walks out the way of the door and catches Andrew up.

I fill my top bowl with some warm water and place some of the wipes inside the water ready for Malcolm. I wheel the bowl out of the sluice room and Valencia follows me like an obedient puppy. I knock on the door to Malcolm's room and enter. Malcolm is fast asleep.

Malcolm is a 94 year old man, who, after fighting in a world war for his country and working his nose to the grindstone in a wood factory, developed vascular dementia eight years ago, meaning that the basic blood supply to his brain is failing. In order to maintain good health and function, brain cells need a good supply of blood. This blood is delivered through blood vessels known as the vascular system. If this area becomes damaged and blood cannot reach the brain, then the brain cells die. This can lead to increased aggression, memory loss, and agitation. Sometimes there can be mini strokes in the brain known as Transient Ischemic attacks (or 'TIA's). This will cause further damage to the blood vessels and ultimately the brain. If that wasn't enough already, we were also rewarding Malcolm, by getting him up out of his bed at 8.15am.

Now as a student and ultimately as a qualified nurse you work to a specific code of practice governed by the Nursing and Midwifery Council (NMC), and at the heart of all this means that the patient must always come first, and you must try to abide by their decisions and preferences. I'm not a mind reader, but I'm wondering how many 94 year old men would want to be made to get up at 8:15am every morning?

As I get closer to Malcolm who is still fast asleep, I feel myself saying the words that all the other nurses have said. I hate myself for saying it, but the words just continue to come out, as I gently place a hand on Malcolm's shoulder. 'Malcolm, time to get up, it is time for your breakfast Malcolm'. Malcolm stirs. 'What?, what!' . 'Malcolm', I gently rock him again. Malcolm opens his eyes briefly. 'What do YOU want, just leave me be for five minutes!'.

I look at Valencia who is looking at me with a kind of fixed blank stare, awaiting her next instruction. I want to leave Malcolm, but I know if I go out of his room and tell Linda that he doesn't want to get up, she will just laugh in my face and tell me I'm not assertive enough. Since when did life become like this? - that we can't let a 94 year old man with dementia get a bit more shut eye. I know it won't work, I almost have to accept that this is the way things are done round here, and either way Malcolm needs to get up. I try again, this time a little louder and instead of patting his arm, I reach towards his shoulder and ask 'Malcolm, we need to help you to stand up and assist you on to the commode please, its breakfast time'.

Malcolm opens his eyes fully now. Malcolm has a very elongated face, and still has some bristling white hair, which is parted away from his balding spot that runs right down the centre of his very spherical forehead. He has a set of yellowing decaying teeth which he is showing me this morning again as he utters and spits out at me.

'LOOK, just leave ME alone I said, leave me be' Malcolm shouts. I keep uttering the same statement over and over. I am gradually able to assist, working with Malcolm to slowly lift him up with the help of Valencia by his feet so that he is sitting on the bed, his arms trying to hit out at us, but I keep his hand in my hand. He is incredibly powerful and has an iron grip which I am constantly having to put pressure on to stop him from punching out at me. 'Malcolm, can you stand with us please, we are going to help you on the toilet'. 'NO YOU'RE FUCKING NOT, I'm going to call the police, get away with you.' Malcolm starts trying to bite at me. I dodge away, I can feel my pristine polo shirt starting to feel slightly damp with sweat. 'MUMMY, MUMMY', Malcolm starts screaming out at us. 'Come on Malcolm, stand with us please.' 'WHAT ?' Malcolm shouts out. I explain it again to him. He looks at me a little puzzled, then at Valencia. 'Oh all right then' he mumbles. We help to stand him up and guide him on the commode. He always seems to calm down a bit once he is sat down on here. I begin undressing his damp pyjama top and bottom. 'What are you doing?' he shouts. 'I'm just helping to take your pyjamas off Malcolm, and we're going to help you into some clean clothes, ready for breakfast. Are you hungry?' 'No, not really' he sighs.

I wheel the bowl around awkwardly on its three wheels, and start dabbing at the water with the wipe, and begin to gently wash Malcolm as best I could. He would be able to wash himself a little with gentle prompting. I think back to the university skills lectures in which we practised this very same routine, but on a plastic dummy. My, how things are different in the real world, they certainly don't teach you about when patients talk back to you and fight!

There is a knock at the door, it's Linda. 'You two OK in here?' Before we can answer she starts speaking again. 'When you have finished with Malcolm you can go get John up, and we need to be quick because we're running late'. She suddenly glances at Valencia who has started to tidy up the remains of Malcolm's bed and starts stripping it for some fresh new sheets. Linda starts up in a very patronising voice with a shrill edge to it 'Didn't we learn anything in manual handling classes then?' She goes over to the bed, and starts pumping the green lever on the bottom of the bed with her foot to raise the bed up higher so that Valencia doesn't have to stoop so low in order to change the bed sheets. 'We don't want any back injuries on this ward thank you very much.' And with that Linda was out the door in a flash. Malcolm, who is still sitting on the commode, looks at me blankly.

'What are we doing then? I want to see him now!' Malcolm orders. 'It's OK Malcolm, we're going to help you to get dressed and ready for breakfast'. We help Malcolm back up and change his pad, which is a feat harder than you think. Changing a grown man's lower extremities can sometimes present itself with quite a challenge, particularly when the man in question is trying to kick and scream, completely confused and agitated as to why you are 'messing' around with his lower half in the first place.

Luckily this morning Malcolm appears to have calmed down a little, and so I am able to get his pants and socks on with relative ease. I look in Malcolm's drawer for some nets. Nets are an incredible invention. They resemble the sort of pants you used to have to wear at school if you had an 'accident' they are incredibly stretchy and are designed to hold in the patient's pad during the day or night. Unfortunately I can only ever seem to find one size on the ward, and that seems to be the super small size, which makes it a task in itself to fit them over a grown man's leg, let alone all the way around his pad. I find the pair of nets and tell Malcolm what I'm about to do. 'What you doing?' Malcolm shouts. 'It's OK Malcolm, I'm just putting your pants on'. Repetition is often needed due to Malcolm's short term memory loss, a common problem with dementia patients. Malcolm seems very uninterested in what I have to say, and who can blame him I think to myself, I have just essentially dragged a 94 year old man out of bed, in order to make sure he fits into the system of having his breakfast at a set time each morning.

I realise I haven't got any trousers out for Malcolm. I look in his wardrobe, and to my despair I cannot see any, except for an old pair of pyjama bottoms. 'Keep an eye on him' I say to Valencia, as I go out the door, in the search for some of Malcolm's trousers. I catch Andrew on the way confidently wheeling his bowls to the next patient, 'Hey, where are Malcolm's trousers?' I realise afterwards this is a fairly ridiculous question to be asking, but it's too early in the morning for me to think that clearly, so I just go ahead and ask it anyway. Andrew stares at me blankly. 'If there aren't any in his wardrobe, you will just have to get some from stores'. 'Stores!' I cry out, 'so basically I have to dress a 94 year old mentally ill man in some random clothes?' 'What else do you want me to do? If there are no clothes, then there are no clothes, laundry is coming later this afternoon'. 'Great', I utter, just great, I think to myself. Andrew shrugs at me and continues on confidently wheeling his bowl trolley.

Stores is like a graveyard for clothes. Just like in school you had those special pants when there was a particular incident, or those spare gym kits you wished didn't exist when you had the cunning plan of 'forgetting' your gym kit on gym day. The stores were like a mish mash of clothing from the end of time itself. A lot of the patients who died on the ward were big contributors to the stores cupboard, and who knows where all the other clothing came from, because there was a very interesting mix of clothes right back to what looked like war time clothing. I couldn't believe I was spending my time trying to guess what size trousers Malcolm would require. There wasn't much choice either, the stores cupboard had been randomly organised too. There seemed to be a mix of female and male clothing, and some big fake fur coats pushed all the way to the back, there was hardly any room in here too, and just a pile of odd socks randomly strewn across the floor. I manage to find some pale blue trousers with a pull cord. These would just have to do. I walk out of the cupboard and back to Malcolm's room. Malcolm is still sat on the commode clutching Valencia's hand. He looks at me as I walk in, but does not utter a word.

I pull the trousers up around Malcolm's ankles, then Valencia and I gradually help Malcolm to stand up. Malcolm has become a lot calmer whilst I have been away it seems. We pull up his trousers, and manage to somehow squeeze the net pants up and around his pad, and pull the trousers tight. There is a two inch gap from the bottom of the trousers to Malcolm's ankles. 'Great' I utter to myself, hoping that Malcolm's son wouldn't come and visit him today, and see what a shambles we had made of his father's clothing.

Valencia and I manage to get Malcolm's slippers on, and slowly stand him up, and walk with him outside of his room, and help to sit him down on a chair outside. Malcolm quickly goes back to sleep, and Valencia finishes up tidying the rest of the room. I still feel incredibly hot, and look down at my watch; 8.35am. This was going to be a long day indeed, I could feel it.

I wheel the bowl back to the sluice room, awkwardly. The wheel turns right around, and the water suddenly goes flying up in the air and splashes all over the floor. Just what I needed, I hated these damn trolleys, today was just getting better and better.

Linda rushes past me. 'Don't forget to do John's BM'S either will you'. 'No', I say through clenched teeth. John's blood sugar levels needed to be taken each morning, as he was an insulin dependent diabetic. His levels had to be carefully monitored. The normal range for a diabetic should be between 4-7mmols. Anything drastically higher or lower than these values could cause John to go into a coma and ultimately a risk of death. Being either hypoglycaemic (low blood sugar) or hyperglycaemic (high blood sugar) was something very dangerous, so they were not to be taken lightly. What this meant for me was that I had to get a tiny digital machine out from the drugs room, and a tiny lancet, and gently prick John on his finger, which was a task that was harder than it seemed, for John didn't like it one bit, and often flailed around wildly with his hands hitting out at whoever was trying to get the reading from him. You needed just enough blood for the machine to whir into gear. Excruciatingly at times you would almost get enough blood, but not quite enough to trigger the machine, which meant getting another needle and starting the procedure all over again.

John was another 90 year old gentleman, but he posed a bigger challenge than Malcolm, as he was bed and chair bound. He needed to be hoisted up into his chair for mealtimes. This meant utilising the wards new hoist machine and hoping that it had batteries and was fully operational. Despite being new it had broken down last week, and thus a large calamity had ensued as John was still winched high in the air when it had failed, which meant all the nursing team were running around and trying to work out if there was a manual override, whilst John was left two foot in the air in the hoist shouting blue murder at everyone demanding that they got him down. Luckily there was a spare battery in the office, and the situation was calmed down quickly afterwards. The hoists usually worked well, and resembled being strapped into a small sling chair which could then be raised and lowered and positioned to your liking, the advantage being you could hoist patients up off the floor or from their bed if needed. I always felt a little awkward using any machinery, as there always seemed too many straps and clips to them, but you soon got used to them, especially after training using them on a daily basis. They just became part of the routine.

I walk into John's room. The door was already open as Valencia had gone in before me with a freshly cleaned new bowl of warm water. John was trying to entice her close to him and his arms were flailing about wildly. You had to be careful with John, as he could frequently hit out at you and try to punch or scratch. 'Come here you, COME HERE'. Valencia was stuck rigid, refusing to get any nearer. 'Hi JOHN,' I say in my best nursing voice I can muster (two parts enthusiasm, with one part assertion). John was very deaf, so I had to speak very loudly and clearly at every stage. Linda suddenly appears from nowhere. 'What are his bm's?' 'I haven't done them yet' I state clearly. 'Well I need to know, and when you have done them can you record them in the charts please'. 'Sure', I say. Linda just doesn't leave me alone, I barely have time to breathe when she is on duty. I see Andrew walking up the corridor past John's door. 'I'm going to get breakfast ready, OK?' 'yeh sure, we're just getting John up, and then is that it?' 'Yes think that's everyone after that, no problem', Andrew smiles and saunters up the corridor in a confident manner. I still wonder how he can keep up the smiles and the confidence day in day out. I make a mental note to ask him this later on.

I found out from past experience that it's best to just be as quick as possible when getting John's blood sugars. I had everything ready in my hand so I just walked up to John, and stated clearly what I was going to do. You have to always be informing your patients of what you are going to do to them. I lightly grabbed his left hand and made a small pin prick. Luckily enough blood trickled into the sensor on the machine, I then had to wait twenty seconds to get a reading...8.8mmols. Not too bad at all considering the previous night it was apparently up to 20.5mmols. Myself and Valencia slowly work on getting John into the hoist. This involves a lot of rolling John gently to and fro to get a hoist underneath him and secure him tightly onto the machine. The hoist is quite a scary looking device with lots of bars and wheels on, but it does the job, we winch John safely into his chair like an expert JCB driver, and I wheel John up to the dining area, where a lot of the other patients are gathering. The hoist must be quite a traumatic experience for John, well anyone really. As students we actually tried sitting in the hoists and being picked up and put onto a bed in the training rooms of our University building, and even we all felt a little uncomfortable and anxious in them, and we don't have dementia. Andrew is enthusiastically pouring tea and coffee for the patients. I glance at my watch; 8.55am. Time for breakfast at last.

9am – 11am

There are a few patients gathered around the dining area. John is still hitting out at the air in the corner of the room. He waves over to me, beckoning me to come. 'Come here' he shouts. I wonder over to him and I am careful to stand just behind him in case he tries to punch out at me again.

'I say fella, help me out would you', he mumbles.

'What is it you need John ?'

'I say help me out fella, move me along' John utters.

'Move you where John ?'

'Move me up the chair would you'. I gently help push him up the chair so he is sat up straighter, ready for breakfast. I adjust the pillow behind him and he smiles at me for a brief moment.

Suddenly the alarm goes, it's the front door, the alarm goes off as soon as it is opened just to alert the staff each time in case it is a patient who has managed to escape the clutches of the ward. It pays to be careful, and security is of paramount importance on this ward, where people are extremely vulnerable.

Andrew is preparing breakfast for everyone, there is a standard choice of cornflakes, porridge or weetabix. I smile as I see a menu up on the wall offering a much larger and varied choice of breakfast for each day of the week. Those days are long gone. The menu was even encased in a glass frame, and had pictures to highlight some of the food on offer.

'Can you make the tea and coffee please?' Andrew beckons to me. One of the biggest problems I always had was trying to remember exactly which patient had what drink, and whether they were diabetic or not. Some of the patients would be able to tell me exactly what they wanted, but others I had to just try and remember. Usually it was fine. I started pouring out the tea, usually just half way and then filled the rest of the cups up with milk, as to make them luke warm. You never know when you are going to get a cup of tea thrown at you, so best to be prepared and make it as safe as possible for you and the patient. I walk over to Liz, a small and very frail old lady with white hair. She has an arched back which has a large lump on it, like a hunchback, which has caused her considerable pain in the past, but now she is on Matrifen pain relief patches which slowly releases the drug gradually over a period of 72 hours. She has brilliant white hair, and reminds me of my nan who has been dead for over five years now. She even came from the same area of Birmingham my nan was bought up in. I ask her what she wants to drink. 'Tea please love', and she smiles at me, 'how much will that be love ?', I explain it's free, she looks at me very confused. 'Are you sure love?'

'Yes, it's quite all right' I reply, 'it's completely free!' She pauses for a moment.

'You are good to me aren't you love'. She smiles at me again. I go and get the cup of tea for her and return with it. She smiles. 'That's smashing thank you, ooh, it looks a proper nice cup of tea that!', and she takes it off me, continuing to smile.

I finish up making the drinks. It is just me and Andrew still in the lounge area. Andrew whispers over to me.

Andrew: 'Hey man, what do you make of that Valencia?'

Jack: 'She's OK,' I reply.

Andrew: 'Fantastic body on her you know, she's lovely, I'd love to show her some extra special attention'.

Andrew: 'Would you like any toast, there's some spare if you like, just remember to stand in the corner so you don't get seen by any management.'

Jack: 'Yeah sure no problems, do you want any?'

Andrew: 'No, I am fine thank you.'

There was an unwritten rule in the hospital that once all the patients had been fed, the staff were able to help themselves to some porridge or cereal or a few rounds of toast. The official rule is that you were not allowed, and if any management caught you then you could be in some serious trouble. The kitchen however was quite spacious and there was a corner in which you could stand away from the windows in which you would not be seen by any outside people walking past. What usually happened is we would take it in turns to make our toast, and whoever was in the lounge would keep a watch out for anyone coming onto the ward from the main entrance. This usually meant you were in a hurried state of stressful eating, but without a few rounds of toast, the day seemed to drag that little bit longer, so it was always useful to grab the odd snack whilst you could.

Andrew walked into the kitchen whilst I was still attending to my toast.

Andrew: Hey, what do you make of that other student nurse we have here? Now she is nice, for an older lady.

Jack: You're a man obsessed!

Andrew: I just like my women. I remember when I worked at the kebab shop, you always had so many to choose from I'm telling you, wow I miss those days.

Jack: How long did you work there?

Andrew: About a year, always trouble with drunk people though, although what we used to do if some of the lads gave us trouble and asked for chilli sauce we always put the fiercest sauce we'd got on there, and you could see sometimes they would be crying into their kebabs, we always had the last laugh.

I start eating my toast. Andrew is cleaning the last few bits and pieces up. There is a large white plastic bucket where all the remains of the uneaten porridge and toast is thrown into. Sometimes looking at it just makes me feel a little queasy, it's like a proper 'slop' bucket.

Once I finish my toast and have a cup of coffee, I feel a little happier and charged up. It's just gone half past ten. The next task of the day was to toilet the patients. Most were not able to walk themselves and most needed at least two people to help take them to the toilet. Of all the tasks of the day toileting could be quite a traumatic experience depending on the patient. It sounds a fairly simple task, but you would never know what to expect sometimes. Andrew and I went to see Martin, an 85 year old man who was suffering from Korsakoff's syndrome, an alcohol induced dementia. Martin had been a real bad boy in his past, stealing cars, robbery, and he even tried to set his house on fire with his mother still in the building. He couldn't speak very well, but when he did speak sort of came out with a whisper, and he could get very agitated and aggressive if you didn't understand what he was saying. He was of medium build, and he reminded me of Jack Nicholson in terms of his receding hair line and sometimes maniacal grin. Often, at the start of a shift, Martin would be in the lounge area, reading a newspaper with his thick black shades on. He would wave to me if he saw me, and soon get back to his paper. I liked Martin, he wasn't particularly aggressive although you did have to watch for his agitation sometimes, on the whole you could converse a little with him, and play some basic board games with him, and card games. Myself and Andrew approached Martin and asked him if he would like to go to the toilet. He nodded, and stood up, he just needed a little guidance sometimes so we both walked him into the toilet.

The usual procedure was helping Martin take his trousers and pants down, removing his pad, and sitting him down on the toilet. Sometimes running the tap in the sink helped remind dementia patients where they were and orientated them to the time and place. Martin would have varying amounts of insight but generally he seemed to understand where he was and what purpose to carry out. We sat him down and Andrew turned to Martin.

Andrew: You're on the toilet Martin OK, you do what you have to please, and we will be here to help if you need it.

Martin nodded. After a few short moments he starting straining a little, he gestured his hand towards mine, he wanted to hold it.

After a few moments more, and a lot more squeezing, Martin looked a lot more relieved and less red in the cheeks. I asked if he had finished, he nodded, we helped him up off the toilet, cleaned him up, put a fresh pad on him, pulled his trousers up, and I was about to flush the toilet when..

I noticed Martin had filled the toilet bowl.

I flushed the toilet...

The toilet whirred into gear, the water level rose a little, but this deposit wasn't going to go down, Martin had effectively blocked the toilet!

'It's not going down,' I say to Andrew.

Andrew: 'It's what!'

Jack: 'It's just not flushing'

Martin is oblivious to the situation that is developing.

Jack: 'Someone's going to have to get it out.'

There was a large pause. I thought to myself there is no way on earth I can attempt something like this, the smell and the thought of having to try and clean it out was already making me feel a little queasy, then all of a sudden Andrew launched into action, he grabbed a white plastic apron, scrunched it up in his hand, and turned to me.

Andrew: 'It's OK, I've seen shit a million times, let me just scoop it out and put it in the bin, no problems'

And then without flinching Andrew just stuck his hand into the toilet bowl and started scooping it up with his hands in the plastic apron and throwing it into the bin beside the sink. I couldn't believe my eyes, by now the smell had filled the entire toilet, and I was starting to feel a little sick, but Andrew seemed to be on a mission and in some ways seemed to be strangely enjoying the challenge. After a few good scoops, Andrew flushed the toilet and everything else vanished down the bowl. We walk outside with Martin and show him to a seat.

Andrew: 'All in a day's work'

'Yeah', I mutter, and think of a nice tranquil beach in my head. I think to myself, could the day get any crazier?

Once everyone had been toileted, it was really a case of trying to entertain or get involved with activities until lunchtime.

11am – 1pm

What usually happened next was an attempt to find something that was actually complete and undamaged in the activities cupboard. I decided to go and have a look in the cupboard for anything that might be at all suitable. Inside the cupboard were bits of old crayons, old biscuit tins with lots of random brushes and paints in, and an assortment of playing cards seemed to be strewn across most of the shelves. Towards the end of the cupboard on the floor were a large pile of jigsaws. I decided to grab the nearest one to me, a wildlife jigsaw puzzle, a 100 piece. I would often try and get the patients involved in doing a jigsaw puzzle, most really appreciated the distraction to the ward, and often you could have a chat with some of the patients whilst doing them. Many of the staff didn't seem to like the 'clutter' of a jigsaw remaining on the tables and would often hurriedly pack it away when your back was turned even before it was completed! I grabbed the jigsaw and took it back out into the lounge and placed it on the table. Before I could do anything else I started to hear some banging and some shouts.

'HELP, HELP, ROGER, ROGER!'. Another huge thud. I rushed around to the corridor, to see Liz with her frame in her hand smashing it against the window and shouting out at the top of her voice.

'ROGGGEERRRR'

I warily approached her.

Jack: Liz, what's the matter?

Liz: Get out! I want my Roger, he is supposed to be coming to see me.

Roger was Liz's husband and visited fairly regularly to see Liz, but she would frequently get upset or confused as to where she was at times, and would get quite agitated like just now.

Liz: Where is he?!

Jack: He might be coming to see you later, Liz.

Liz: I want to see him now, where is he, and you get out my house!

Jack: Liz, Roger will visit you later today after lunch sometime, please stop banging on the window.

Liz: I will bang on this window all I fucking want to!

She proceeded to bang on the window, she then walked closer up to the window and started to try and peer outside of the window. Because of her height she had to go on tiptoes to fully see outside of the window. She started crying.

Liz: I just want to see my Roger, look he only lives over there.

She pointed to an old church within the grounds of the hospital which was only a few minutes walk away.

Jack: Liz, he doesn't live there, that's an old church.

Liz: You're a fucking liar you are, he lives there, and why won't you let me see him, he wants to come here but you won't, please let me out, why wouldn't you let me out to see him?

She starts to tap lightly on the window as someone walks past, it's almost like she has realised the futility of her situation and is gradually losing the will power and energy to fight against it. Unfortunately we really were keeping her in here, but it was for her own good. She posed a specific risk to herself and others, sectioned under the Mental Health Act under section 3, which meant we could keep her here for treatment for up to 6 months, and work towards her best interests with regard to her medication regime. Whether it's morally acceptable or not this is how the act works, and the key elements are always risk, to self or others. I did feel sorry for her, but she just didn't have capacity to understand that she was at risk to herself and from falling if she was to go home and live with her husband, Roger. In fact it was Roger himself who found he couldn't cope with Liz's behaviour any longer, he was getting stressed out himself and was very upset. It is often a massive impact on families and friends when a loved one develops an illness of this kind.

Liz: Please tell me where my Roger is and let me out!

Jack: I'm sorry, I can't let you out I'm afraid, you're in a hospital, Roger will visit you later.

Liz: I am NOT in a hospital! This is my house!

Jack: Come and sit down in the other room, and I'll get you a cup of tea.

Liz: NO! I'm staying here till my Roger gets here.

I decided to leave Liz at the window. She was clearly agitated and quite aggressive, so it wasn't worth trying to persuade her to go into another room whilst she appeared quite hostile.

As I walked into the lounge area there were still a few patients sitting around. Malcolm was still there but he seemed a little anxious. One of the carers had wedged him tightly into his chair and then stuck him right up close underneath the table so that it was very difficult for him to get out. This was a common trick in this hospital, whether it was a lack of staff or a lack of caring, no patient should be held against their will.

I went over to see Malcolm, he was waving me over.

Malcolm: Hey, will you help me?

Jack: Sure, what would you like Malcolm ?

Malcolm: Well, I want to get out of here!

Jack: OK sure, let's go for a walk.

I help Malcolm up from his chair, and just slowly walk around the corridor a little with him, and try to calm him down. It will soon be lunch time, he was a little unsteady on his feet but able to walk with a little assistance from me.

I walked past the office. Linda had just come off the phone, and shouted over to me

Linda: Hey luvee, I need you to book transport later, and do some care plans, you should be able to do that, shouldn't you, as a third year student?

Her tone was as condescending as ever. I decided not to let it get to me and just answer back as normal.

Linda: Oh and I also need you to change Stan's colostomy bag, that will be fun for you.

Typical, I just knew she wanted a reaction out of me for that, I had never changed a colostomy bag before, but I could tell from Linda's tone that she was just waiting for a groan off me or a disgruntled look, but I gave it my best confident manner and just said that would be no problem and I would sort it. This day was going to be a long one, that was for sure. I looked at my watch, it was almost time for lunch, I had to start getting people back and ready to sit at the table. I turned Malcolm round slowly and started heading back towards the lounge, already I could hear the movement of chairs and the food trolley clanking about.

1pm – 3pm

Lunch time was usually fairly routine. Most people were escorted gently to the chairs, and everyone most of the time sat around in a fairly orderly fashion. Andrew was rushing around as usual making sure everyone was furnished with fresh plastic cups and beakers. Andrew knew the routine almost too well. I'd never seen someone work so fast, and be so enthusiastic in his job. We are standing by the drinks trolley waiting for the main food trolley to be wheeled in and plugged in. You could hear these trolleys every day, clanking about as the men and women wheeled them out to each and every ward, large steel boxes on wheels housing the most interesting and brightly coloured food items. Usually the 'feeds', for those patients who could not swallow very well or had difficulty with large items of food, and would normally be treated to very soft mush. Sometimes it would be hard to tell what was a main meal and what was pudding due to the colour combinations the kitchen staff had created (with the help of lots of E numbers no doubt). Andrew started to tell me another story about when he used to work for the kebab shop in town.

One of the male kitchen staff soon arrives with the food trolley, he manoeuvres it smoothly into the corner of the room, plugs it in, and with a nod, he disappears. He does this every single day, exactly the same mannerisms, at exactly the same time.

Andrew begins to prepare the feed meals. My role here is usually to feed the patients who need help the most and cannot feed themselves. Due to the nature of the dementia a lot of physical control has now gone, sometimes there is a faint flicker of a memory of what to do when their meal is placed in front of them, but as dementia largely affects short term memory, by the time some of the patients have picked up a knife or fork they have forgotten what to do with it. Some success can be found in giving little 'cues' and tapping the knife or fork against the dish so as to serve as an auditory cue, but for the most part there are a number of patients who need feeding every single day. Andrew prepares me a fresh plate of lightly brown coloured mixture, with some white fluffy pieces (which I assume to be potato), and some bright luminous green mixture (which I assume to be peas).

I go over to a patient known as Kevin. Kevin used to be a bus driver, he has been in this ward for about five years now, he's still quite young, in his mid 60s, and occasionally you can get a glimmer of what Kevin used to be like behind his cold brown eyes. The odd responses are few and far between but sometimes you will get some response or a wry smile. A lot of people describe dementia as robbing the real person, and a lot of people can have quite a vacant look. Speaking to the patients' relatives can often give you a much broader picture of what they used to be like, but I will never see that, so I can only imagine. It is here when you think what a cruel illness dementia can be, although we can only hope that the patients no longer have much of an insight into their illness and are hopefully not suffering with the knowledge of what is going on.

I sit down with Kevin, and begin spooning the food into his mouth. He gives me a small smile, a flash of recognition maybe. Kevin can be quite hard to feed as he often gets up from the table and wanders up and down the corridor on the unit, often for hours and hours at a time, even at lunchtime. Often the signals for feeling hungry are not transmitted up to the brain any more. Rather than forgetting to eat, your brain hasn't actually told you that you are even hungry, which is why it is so important to be feeding Kevin in this manner. Today Kevin seems to remain much more settled. I continue to use my auditory cues and tap at the bowl, sometimes trying to let Kevin put the spoon in his own hand and let him try to feed himself. I often try to do this so at least to try and give back at least some autonomy to the patients, and let them feel in control, although of course it is not always possible. Sitting next to Kevin is an 85 year old gentleman known as Derek. Derek is the most vocal person I have ever come across, and will often be shouting and raising his fist to anyone that comes near him. Sometimes I will get a soldier's salute from him, but other times Derek will come out with the most foul mouthed insults almost continuously. Derek is looking over in my direction, he has spotted a plastic beaker full of tea which is destined for Kevin. He starts pointing at the beaker whilst looking at me.

Derek: Hey sir! Give us a go on that will you? Go on, give us a go.

Jack: It's OK, your tea is coming in a minute Derek.

Derek: Oh FUCK OFF! Give us a go on that will you, you CUNT!

This was the normal language for Derek most lunchtimes. At first it was quite difficult to get used to, bad language is common in mental health, but it was best to sort of let it sail over you and just get on with the job in hand. I carried on feeding Kevin, and eventually Derek was given his own beaker of tea and his lunch. Derek was capable of feeding himself, but sometimes he would like to steal other people's food as well as his own, so it was always a good idea to keep an eye on what he was doing from time to time. I had finished feeding Kevin so I went up to Andrew to get him some pudding. Whilst I was doing this I suddenly heard Derek shouting again.

Derek: You cunt!

I looked over my shoulder, and Derek with his fork in his hand was waving it in Kevin's face. Kevin hadn't taken kindly to this and had grabbed hold of Derek's hand and wouldn't let go, so they were both locked together. I instantly ran over to try and separate them. I stood right in the middle of them and managed to push Derek's hand away from Kevin's. I was just about to walk back and get Kevin's pudding when all of a sudden, Kevin started trying to punch and kick out at me. I immediately had the kick of adrenalin involved with my flight or fight response and ran down towards the corridor out of the way. Kevin immediately stood up and all of a sudden his usual walking pace had suddenly turned into more of a running sprint, he pointed at me and shouted 'YOU'. I ran straight down the corridor, passing Linda and the student nurse who were in the office. I thought they would have offered some support in this instance, but once they had realised what was going on I could hear them laughing about what had just happened, I guess the sight of me running down the corridor would have been fairly amusing, but I was genuinely quite scared. I reached the bottom of the corridor, and took a few moments to pause and think things through, Kevin had seemingly forgotten about the situation as I could already see that he had turned around and was walking back towards the lounge area. I walked slowly back, passing the office in which the student nurse and Linda were still in hysterics. I glanced at them, smiled and carried on towards the lounge. I found Kevin wandering and sat him down, not next to Derek this time. Andrew handed me his pudding and I started again. Andrew was also smiling to himself.

Andrew: You moved quick eh man!

I grin at Andrew. My adrenalin levels were tailing off a bit. As I carried on feeding Kevin, he had seemingly forgotten about the whole incident that had just happened and continued to give me the odd grin and widened eyes when I asked him to eat a little bit more of his pudding. Eventually everyone had been fed, and Andrew was hurriedly rushing around cleaning up everyone's plates and cups and putting them back on the food trolley so it could be collected. There were a few trays of chips left over so Andrew conveniently put them in the kitchen area, out of the way, so that we could walk into the kitchen to do something else, and steal the odd chip as we were carrying on with our work, out of sight of any managers who may be on the prowl. Linda walks into the kitchen not long after I have deposited a rather large mouthful of chips in my mouth.

Linda: Luvee don't forget it's ward round in an hour or so, so I hope you have got everything ready for that, and that you know what you are saying, have you got all the weekly reviews ready?

Jack: Yeah most of them, I'll sort that in a minute.

Linda: Well get on with it won't you? You know Dr Bauenbacker doesn't suffer fools gladly, and he will expect everything there for him, he is a very busy man you know.

Jack: Yeah I know.

Dr Bauenbacker; I had heard his name before meeting him, his legendary status has become apparent throughout the whole of the hospital building, a 50 something suave and sophisticated doctor. A doctor who knows he is good, and can get away with turning up in fresh cream trousers and sandals, he sports a thick wavy mane of silver hair, and he often sweeps it back with his hand. His ward rounds were often legendary. I hadn't been to many, but the ones I had attended could be more bizarre than your day's work. The first time I met him I actually thought he was one of the patients, the way he was acting. He was very condescending towards students in particular, so I was not looking forward to leading a ward round with him. The ward round basically meant I had to summarise what had gone on with each patient for the week, any particular changes in behaviour, how they were eating and drinking, and how they were responding to their medication, and any other matters that may need discussing such as social worker input and suitability for discharging out into the community. The doctor would usually have a trainee doctor with him, someone he could bark his orders out to and generally test his knowledge on medication. This time I was not going to have any help, I was going to lead the ward round myself. It shouldn't be too difficult though, nothing much had happened in the week, and I was fairly confident. Most of the time it would just be a case of summarising. The only thing you would have to sometimes watch out for is if Bauenbacker was on some sort of a mission to humiliate and could often ask quite awkward questions, which could be quite embarrassing, especially if any patients' relatives were in the room and a full team of social workers and occupational therapists. There was nothing I could do about it, Linda was firmly set on me being launched into everything today as I was a 'third year student' and she just loved to keep reminding me of this, but I wouldn't break. Not today. Not any day when she was on. You could just tell she was waiting for me to give her a sarcastic or angry response back, but no, I had decided I was going to play this one cool. This was one student she was not going to break, no matter what she tried to throw at me.

I help Andrew finish off wiping the tables down. Most of the patients are sat now in more comfortable chairs, some in front of the T.V in the other living area. I walk into the office and begin getting out all of the files for the patients, and begin extracting the weekly review sheets from each one. I start by making notes of anything I wish to say about each patient, if anything is pressing or needs discussing from the previous week. Some patients have had considerable social worker input, and some are still needing to be placed elsewhere such as a nursing home, so these are all relevant details that will need discussing and chasing up.

It is often fascinating looking through the large bound notes of each patient. Most are actually bursting to the seam with all sorts of medical history and personal background, often it is quite sad though, and you can get quite an accurate picture of what this person was like growing up and all the hospital admissions they have had throughout their years. As I sit here in the office sometimes I think of these people's lives and it often reminds me how I should make sure that I try to lead a good and fulfilled life, because there is no closer reminder working within this area of mental health about how short and precious life is, and how often it is often cut short with drastic consequences, so in a way I guess it can be a gift, it can make you live out all your dreams and accomplish everything you set out to do, but on the other hand I guess it can sometimes be a permanent reminder of potentially what you yourself could be heading for, or indeed a member of your family, or one of your friends. It is difficult sometimes, and I cannot count the amount of times a patient's family member has come up to me and said 'I don't know how you can do it', or 'how do you cope with it day in day out?' I guess you have to be a certain type of person, patience is certainly a virtue, you need lots of it, but everyone is human at the end of the day, and people's patience will eventually run out. Maybe we have a higher tolerance and can accept what we do day in day out, but it certainly isn't easy, particularly not as a student.

As a student you are somewhere in between the real world and the fake world. The world of academia and essays is a comfortable zone away from the harsh realities of life on the ward, but on qualifying, that will all disappear, something I am realising all too well as I step foot on this ward each day. My days are numbered, no longer will I be able to hold the title of student nurse, and one day I won't be able to say 'sure, I'll just get the nurse for you', I will be that nurse! I will need to get on and deal with things. I look at the clock, its almost 3pm, Dr Bauenbacker usually turns up around now. I go back to my notes and make sure I have everything in order.

Linda walks into the office and alerts me that the doctor is here with his associate, and that they are in the far room on the right. She smiles at me, one of those horribly false smiles again, and I smile back equally as fake and thank her for the information. She walks off in the direction of the lounge calling after the other student nurse that she has currently got taking everybody's blood pressure even though I did everyone's this morning, and they are usually only taken once a day. Her luck was in today as she had two student nurses she could try and control. The other student nurse also didn't seem to be showing any signs of giving in and was fulfilling all the tasks that Linda had been setting her throughout the day.

I gather my final scraps of paper together and all the weekly review sheets and walk towards the room. I knock on the door and enter. It was a more crowded room than usual. Dr Bauenbacker was there with his associate whom I had not met before, he had long curly black hair and looked to be in his mid 20's, he was wearing an immaculate plain white shirt, the top button open revealing a very small silver rope chain around his neck. Dr Bauenbacker was sat next to him, legs crossed, and with a small black biro in his mouth he continued to chew on as he looked up at me, there was another lady in the room with short black hair, and small round silver rimmed glasses. I had met her before, she was a social worker, and she had seemed quite friendly. In her lap she had a huge stack of paperwork, and a black leather diary to her side on the seat. The room was considerably cramped, even with just us four in it, there was a bookcase to the right of the door, and a small desk and computer, with a few seats and sofa surrounding it, this was intended to be the 'students' study area'. I had not managed to spend too much time in here, usually thanks to Linda barking her orders at me, but usually you could grab a few minutes in here if you wanted to do some research and get on with some of your assignments. This was not something that was usually accepted by the university, being on placement and doing your university work was a bit of a grey area. As a student you are not supposed to be counted in the numbers of the general working staff, thereby achieving 'supernumery status', you should be allowed at key times to be able to study for assignments and general reflective writing (writing about events that you had been involved with that you thought were important or highlighted as key areas of learning that would help you progress with your understanding and knowledge base of the nursing process). Supernumerary status in reality never really happened much though. Frequently this hospital was very understaffed and you would find yourself being counted as one of the numbers most days, which on the whole wasn't really a problem, although you could sometimes benefit with being able to 'step out' of the ward environment now and again and have some time away to conduct some research. As I was in the third year and this was my final placement, the chances were getting slimmer. I was being prepared to make the big leap from student nurse to staff nurse! And here was the evidence in all its glory, leading the ward round, being in charge and responsible for informing the team of what I thought. I was very nervous though, and wasn't exactly looking forward to the next half an hour or so, but it was too late to turn back, I had to just carry on with it, and just see what I could do, be cool and calm in my thoughts I tried thinking to myself as I sat down in a chair directly opposite Dr Bauenbacker.

Dr Bauenbacker was originally born in Germany, and still had a very thick German accent when he spoke to you, most notably he would sort of hold on to his 'Rights', by making them long and drawn out, so they would be more sounding like 'Riiiiiiggghhhht'. And the amount of times he used to use the word 'wonderful' (although sounding like wunnderful) was just too many to count. If it wasn't a pen in his hand, it would be the tips of his thick black glasses which he also used to suck on and chew, especially when he was thinking of the correct medication or plan for a patient. His associate looked quite nervous, I guess we were going to be in for a fun half an hour. Bauenbacker cleared his throat.

Bauenbacker: Riiighht, is everyone here then?

Jack: Yes, I think so.

Bauenbacker: OK, now do we know everyone, this is my associate (Points to his sidekick on his right hand side) Doctor Dolly, and I think we have met Pamela, the social worker, haven't we all ?

Jack: Yes.

Bauenbacker: And you're the student, aren't you?

I refrain from pointing to my very obvious pristine white polo shirt with the university logo on it and my blue badge clearly stating 'STUDENT NURSE', and simply utter a meek 'yes'.

Bauenbacker: And you're going to be taking this round are you?

Jack: Yes.

Bauenbacker: Excellent, OK, who is first then?

Jack: Shall we start with Malcolm?

Bauenbacker: Malcolm Wilde, OK, yes.

Jack: OK, well, Malcolm has been sleeping well, good diet and fluid intake, however we have noticed that his aggression seems quite apparent in the morning time, and he is quite resistive to hands on care.

Bauenbacker: OK, and what do we feel about that?

Jack: Well, in all honesty I think it would probably be a good idea if we let him sleep in a little, he obviously doesn't like getting dragged out of bed at 8am each morning.

Bauenbacker stares intently at me, quizzical, as though I had said something that had really confused him. He frowns for a few seconds, then looks at Dr Dolly.

Bauenbacker: What medication is he on?

Dr Dolly frantically leafs through a load of paperwork and finds Malcolm's drug chart.

Dolly: Trazadone (anti depressant), aspirin dispersible, lactulose solution (treatment for constipation), and risperidone.

Bauenbacker: OK, how much risperidone is he on?

Dolly: 500mg BD (this meant twice a day). Risperidone is an anti psychotic typically used to treat schizophrenia.

Bauenbacker: Right, lets up the risperidone to 1g BD, thank you Doctor Dolly.

Dr Dolly starts crossing out the drug chart and altering the amount to be given.

I foolishly try and ask for the real justification of this move.

Jack: Should we not maybe be looking at non medical interventions first?

The room goes quiet, Doctor Dolly doesn't look up from his drugs chart, but his pen stops writing.

The silence lasts for what appears to be a whole minute. Bauenbacker doesn't even look in my direction and just announces to the room.

Bauenbacker: Monitor the increase in risperidone and evaluate next week thank you.

And that was it, the final word on the matter, I couldn't believe it, of all the things I have been taught in university, just seemed to be for nothing. Dr Dolly had finished his scribing, Bauenbacker immediately takes the drug sheet out of Dr Dolly's hands and inspects it. He glances for a few seconds, then frowns, and hands it back to Doctor Dolly.

Bauenbacker: Top left hand corner is not crossed out properly, name of drug is spelt incorrectly, correct dosage is not written in its correct box, and alteration has not been dated, thank you.

Dr Dolly realises his mistake, looks a little ashamed and immediately begins scribbling back on the drug chart, hastily looking up at all of us to check whether we had seen all his errors.

Bauenbacker: We will get there soon Dr Dolly, don't worry.

Bauenbacker says this with an air of authority and glee, you could tell he loved being in charge of his associates, really putting them through the mill. I didn't envy Dr Dolly, it was hard enough training to be a nurse, let alone a doctor, I just wouldn't have the brains or patience for it, three years was long enough in my mind to train for anything. I wondered if this was how Dr Dolly got treated wherever he went on every single ward round, in a way it must be a blessing for the doctors to have associates, they just seem to pile on all the work that they don't want to do onto the trainees and let them get on with it. They would be equally accountable for everything their associate did, but you could sense that Bauenbacker almost revelled in his higher power status and just loved to show his associate up in public. I guess that's why you get paid the big money, having to deal with all this added stress. Dr Dolly had finally finished reamending his corrections and passed it straight back to Bauenbacker. Bauenbacker gave it a quick glance over and smiled.

Bauenbacker: Excellent, doctor. OK, who is next?

Jack: next will be Edward Muise, he actually wants to see you himself, shall I go and get him for you?

Bauenbacker: Yes, excellent.

Most of the people on the ward were not able to actually sit in on the ward round and discuss their own issues, but Edward Muise, who was 72, still had enough about him to be able to converse with people and had some insight still left about his welfare and mental health. He had specifically requested to come in to today's ward round. He had been sectioned to this ward on a 136, from the police. A section 136 was the police officer's holding power to move someone from a 'public place' to a place of safety, a prison cell, hospital, etc, if they had reason to believe the person was acting in a manner that appeared to either endanger themselves or others, and appeared to be suffering with mental health problems. Part of the Mental Health Act, this particular section allowed a police officer to remove a person found in a place to which the public have access if he or she believes the person is suffering from a mental disorder and to be in immediate need of care or control. The police officer must consider it necessary to remove the person in their own interests or for the protection of others. Edward had come to this ward as he had become increasingly paranoid about his family wanting to take over his business, most particularly his son. His business was haulage and involved managing a fleet of lorries that would ship construction material all over the country. Edward had built up quite a sizeable business from this single handed, and as old age had crept in he had started letting his son handle some of the finer day to day details and keep up to date with the booking arrangements and accountancy. Most recently there had been reports from the family that Edward had starting acting a little strange during the evenings, locking away large amounts of money in the safe, and displaying paranoid ideas about his son wanting to 'steal the company from him'. There seemed no apparent truth in these ideas, and the family were obviously concerned as to Edward's mental health. The scenario culminated in Edward squaring up to his son one evening as his son was coming back from the office. Edward accused his son of stealing money from him and had started to take a small axe to his son's car, and threatening physical violence to him. His son had no choice but to call the police, and Edward continued to display paranoid thoughts toward his son, so the police felt they had no other option but to enforce the section, took him to a place of safety at the police station and then contacted the hospital. Edward was seen soon after by Dr Bauenbacker, and an approved social worker, his son was also present, and it was deemed necessary to section Edward into care onto this ward, where he has remained for the past week. I got on well with Edward. To look at him you would think he was perfectly fine (and to all intents and purposes he was, this is often an intriguing question most notably asked by most of my friends and family, what does mental health 'look like ?' Any of us can have a mental health problem, we don't all develop reddened eyes and 'menacing looks'.) I often used to chat to Edward in the garden area of the ward, he seemed perfectly pleasant and had plenty of insight, he often used to talk about how he needed to get back to his business and sort his son out before he 'robbed him of everything'. I could only offer a sympathetic ear, in no way could I corroborate with his story, I had no idea if it was true or not. It is quite easy to assume just because people are in hospital then everything they are saying is completely false, but it was not for me to get into, my responsibility was looking after his mental health needs, and giving the best care to him, working on where he was best placed, and if suitable looking at discharging him home with an adequate care package and everything in place to ensure his own safety, and others. Edward always took pride in his appearance, I had seen him earlier today on the ward, he was dressed in black trousers, shoes, and a very crisp black shirt, with silver cuff links. He used to pace around a little up and down the corridor, but would always say hello to me and ask when he could go out into the garden for another chat.

Dr Bauenbacker leans across to me.

Bauenbacker: is there anything we need to know first? What are we looking at here, discharge back home with a care package in place ? (He glances at Pamela)

She takes a few seconds to realise she is being spoken to, rustles a few bits of paper and looks at the doctor.

Pamela: That's right, I have made my assessment, and I have visited the family, they would be happy for a discharge as long as Edward will agree to a visit by us or a member of the community mental health team for at least two weeks.

Bauenbacker: Right, OK, send him in.

I get up off my seat, open the door and go to find Edward. I walk down the corridor, he is normally lying on top of this bed, in his room, staring up at the ceiling. He told me he was bored of this place, and I don't blame him, because of his age he has been sent to this ward, but with as much insight as Edward has it still isn't really the ideal place for him to be, so in that respect he is a bit of an outsider. Most of the other patients here have long lost the ability to speak, so it makes having a conversation very difficult. Edward tries to keep some conversations going with the nursing team and carers, but that isn't always possible as some days we can all be so busy. It seems that there isn't even a minute to spend with the people that should matter the most, our patients. Such is the nature of the industry due to Government staffing levels and financing, a very cynical outlook, but how else can we explain that almost on a daily basis we are constantly ringing nursing agencies to supply us with an extra member of staff, to try and maintain our full quota of two registered nurses and three nursing assistants? In the long run of course this is costing the Government and the hospital a fortune, it must cost at least twice the amount of hiring a care assistant by getting one from the agency, but hey, who am I to argue ? It's out of my control, but I often wonder to myself how constrained 'the system' is. The Government haven't got the money to hire more nurses or care assistants, but the money still has to come from somewhere to pay for all the extra agency help we need! It is a very cynical world we live in, and I often question my motives as it becomes clear that I soon will be no longer a student nurse, but a fully fledged staff nurse, complete and ready to be equally cynical and moan and complain to my colleagues about how were so underpaid and overworked! That scares me a little actually, how you can see yourself becoming someone you really don't want to be, I guess in a way to have that insight can be both a blessing yet a curse. Why should things carry on as they are? Will our mere status as nurses allow us any power to help shift the balance and make things right?

We both walk in through the door, and Edward sits down next to me. Bauenbacker looks across at both of us, leans forward slightly and begins to talk.

Bauenbacker: OK then Edward, how are we doing?

Edward: Well OK I guess, but I could really do with getting back home really and sorting all this out with my son.

Bauenbacker: Riiighhht.

Edward: How long am I going to be kept here?

Bauenbacker looks across at the social worker, she pauses, then begins to speak.

Pamela: Well Edward, I have spoken to the community mental health team, and if you're happy, the care package in place will mean a visit from one of the team twice a day for the first two weeks, and then a follow up visit once a week thereafter. This has been deemed the best course of action, and from speaking to your family they are also in agreement, so it's up to you really.

Edward: And that would mean I could go home today ?

Pamela: Well maybe not today, but if we are all in agreement, I can most probably get the paperwork faxed off and arrange for transport to take you back home tomorrow.

Edward: Right, OK.

Bauenbacker sits upright.

Bauenbacker: Just one thing Edward, how are you getting on with your medication?

Edward: Well, not very well actually, I'm always tired and feel like a walking zombie really, and the one tablet tastes particularly bitter to me.

Bauenbacker: And which one would that be?

Edward: Well it's a very small yellow tablet with a small line down the middle.

Bauenbacker sits back in his chair, and glances over to Doctor Dolly.

Bauenbacker: Risperidone ?

Doctor Dolly looks back at Bauenbacker, and nods his head.

Bauenbacker: Hmmm, I'm not sure about it, what other choices do we have then in the antipsychotics ?

Bauenbacker glances in my direction.

Bauenbacker: Can you get me Edward's Risperidone please?

Jack: Me?

Bauenbacker: Yes please, right away.

I was confused, what was the doctor up to now? I dutifully exit the room, go down the corridor and ask Linda for the keys to the drug cupboard. Linda is just stood in the office, legs and arms crossed, and scowls at me as she hands me the keys.

Linda: Forgot something have we?

Jack: No, it's OK, just something the doctor needs to look at....

Linda: OK, you will get all the summaries done from the ward round once you have finished won't you? They will need to be done before tea, if not then you will just have to stay and do them before you go home tonight, won't you luvee?

Jack: Yeah, no problems.

I walk back down the corridor and open the door to the drugs room. This is where all the patients' drugs are kept, in a locked room, and then in a locked cabinet. At least the drugs were all clearly labelled and all the patients' medication was all in once place, something that wasn't always so organised on some of the other wards. I grab the pack of risperidone tablets, and carefully lock everything back up. As I enter the ward round room again, Bauenbacker immediately sits upright again with his hand outstretched.

Bauenbacker: Ahh , excellent, OK. Dr Dolly, get me the BNF please.

The BNF. British National Formulary, this was the bible for all medications, every student sought one out for free, the price of these were £34.99 if you were to buy them from a reputable bookshop. Published twice a year, it contained absolutely everything you needed to know about all the medications, correct dosage, contra indications, common side effects, and even the price. Many a tale had been told about how students had tried to literally beg borrow and steal these holy gems of information. Rumour had it that the local hospital pharmacy used to dispose of their copies once they got their new ones, but no one was ever quite sure when this was going to take place.

Dr Bauenbacker inspects the box of risperidone, as though he had never seen a package of medication before in his life. After a lot of hmmming and mumbling to himself, he opens the box out, neatly pops a pill out in his hand, licks it a little and then puts it in his mouth. The room falls silent. Dr Bauenbacker has a very quizzical look on his face as he starts crushing and chewing on the tablet in his mouth, you can hear it quite clearly, as this appears to be the only sound going on in the room. Edward looks blankly at Bauenbacker, as does everyone in the room. After much chewing and crumbling later. Dr Bauenbacker sits back quietly for a minute or so, looks at everyone in the room one by one, and then recommences talking.

Bauenbacker: Hmm yes, quite a bit bitter, I see what you mean, what other tablet would you like then?

Edward: Ermm, I'm not quite sure.

Bauenbacker plucks the BNF book from Dr Dolly, and begins leafing through it one by one, and reeling off names of different anti psychotic drugs. After each one is read out, he pauses for a few seconds, looks up at Edward, and waits for Edward's response.

Edward clearly is none the wiser about what any of these drugs do, or indeed how they will taste. Everyone is still reeling from the shocking display by the Doctor, and you could tell everyone wasn't exactly quite sure of how to proceed. Eventually Edward says yes to one of the drugs, I got a sense he just wanted to shut Bauenbacker up and stop this bizarre form of choosing medication. After Edward had decided, Bauenbacker immediately shuts the book up with a sharp snap, sits up and shouts.

Bauenbacker: EXCELLENT! Thank you Edward, you can go now.

Edward looks even more confused, stands up and exits the room. Bauenbacker looks back at me, hands me the box of respiridone, and thanks me. He looks up at his watch, then at Dr Dolly.

Bauenbacker: Righhht, let's keep moving now, time is of the essence.

I continue to look back through my notes of the remaining patients.

I was beginning to think the rumours about Doctor Bauenbacker must all be true. Only last week had I heard that the doctor and the chief medical officer used to give themselves ECT, or Electro Convulsive Shock Treatment. This was usually a last attempt to help anyone with severe depression, for which no medication or psychological therapy had been shown to be working. In the old days it was often quite a barbaric procedure, although in my mind things hadn't changed too much these days. Patients were still wheeled off to a specialist room, given a muscle relaxant and given an electrical current which induced an epileptic seizure. The only way I had ever been told how this works is that it 'shocks the brain' back into gear. Even to this day we are still not quite sure how it works. A doctor essentially sends an electrical current through the brain and tries to recharge it again. I have seen patients make a full recovery after the procedure, and a rapid change in their behaviour and mood, but I have also seen patients missing large parts of their short term memory.

Bauenbacker and the chief medical officer at the time, Brian McGill's, used to be great drinking buddies. Most nights after a shift they would be seen down the local pub drinking merrily away. The pub was a common hang out for a lot of the medical staff at the time.   Mainly trainee doctors, but occasionally some nurses would also be in tow, usually female, and usually in the arms of the trainee doctors. The pub was a strange pub; built in the 1800s, it still had a sort of musty dinginess to it, the main bar area was quite small and compact, leading outside to a rather dull looking beer garden that had a large brick wall surrounding it. On top of this wall was three inch thick barbed wire, that used to remind you of being in a prison ground.   Bauenbacker and Mcgills were completely trashed one night, and decided to sneak back in late to the hospital, and get into the ECT room. McGill's was a 64 year old, stockily built man with a few whispers of grey hair left over his round sunken face. He had a history of depression, and frequently used to have large amounts of time off from the hospital. He had been through two divorces, and subsequently had five children, two from his first marriage, three from his second. They went back to the hospital, into the ECT room, and took it in turns to give each other a quick jolt of electricity to each of their brains. Of course if any of this is true, then they should have been struck off the register in an instant. The strange thing is almost everyone you speak to swears that this is a true story, but of course with no evidence nothing was ever done about it. After today's events I am led to believe that the event may well be true. I also know that Bauenbacker plays golf regularly with the director of the hospital and they are extremely close. There was a strange system going on in this hospital, I think like lots of big companies, a lot of things were built upon 'who you knew' rather than what you knew. Bauenbacker clearly had power, he had been in the business for the past 30 years, and according to many of the females, had eluded all sorts of claims of sexual harassment in the past.   Another rumour claimed he had only got the post in this hospital as the previous hospital he worked at he was forced to resign, due to allegations of harassment of a lot of the junior female doctors. Again, lots of rumours, but no one ever seemed to have any hard hitting evidence about any of these stories ever actually happening.

After getting through the rest of the patients notes, it was pretty plain sailing, and after Doctor Dolly had been suitably reprimanded on almost all of his alterations to the patients' medical notes, it was time for everyone to leave. Before Bauenbacker left, he leans forward again to me.

Bauenbacker: So, what year are you in then?

Jack: Third year, only about three weeks to go actually, then I qualify.

Bauenbacker: Riiighhhhttt, I see.

And with that, Doctor Bauenbacker immediately gets up from his seat, bids me good day, and exits out, with Doctor Dolly and the social worker in tow. They follow him down the corridor like some mini entourage, and they all exit out of the door. I collect my notes together, and carry them all back into the office. There is no one in the office. I glance at the clock; 2:55pm. Maybe I will have some time before tea to get some of these notes written up. There was no sign of Linda, or Valencia, or even the student nurse, whose name I still couldn't remember, despite meeting her at least three or four times already. I couldn't see Andrew, but I could certainly hear him, he was talking to Liz, who thankfully was not trying to smash the hospital windows in with her frame this time.

Andrew: Come here my lovely, here is a wonderful cup of tea for you.

Andrew was shouting this out at the top of his voice. Give him credit, he certainly gained a fantastic rapport with the patients, they smiled at him and he smiled back even more. I quickly walk out the office to see what Andrew is doing, he's doing the drinks round again, this usually happened around now, a cup of tea, and a slice of cake or a biscuit, before the main tea time which would normally come on a trolley again around 5.30pm. Liz is sat down with her walking frame and clutching the cup of tea Andrew has made for her.

Liz: Thank you love, you're a smashing fella, you really are, and handsome.

Andrew: Thank you lovely, you're a lovely lady too.

Liz grins at Andrew and looks a little bashful. She smiles and takes another sip of her tea.

I shout out at Andrew.

Jack: Hey, you need any help Andrew ?

Andrew: No I am fine, thank you anyway, you carry on with your work Mr student nurse!

Jack: OK, no problems.

Andrew looks back at Liz.

Andrew: That man is going to be a new nurse soon, in charge of everything you know.

Liz: Is he now?

Andrew: Yeah, do you like him? He will be responsible for all of this, almost finished his training.

Liz looks at me, smiles, then looks up at Andrew.

Liz: Yes...he's a smashing lad too...

3pm – 5pm

I am sat in the dining area. The faint whispers of family members talking with their loved ones can be heard down the corridor. I hear over the top of this 'If the midget wants to go to bed, then let her!' This bellows out from an 87 year old lady. Her comments are directed at Liz, who is now slowly meandering her way through to the double doors on the other side of the dining area, oblivious to the derogatory comments just shouted at her. You can hear the faint squeak of her walking frame as she passes by. She utters 'How do I get home? Nobody cares!' The lady from the lounge area is still shouting 'LET the midget go to bed!' Her name is Iona.

Liz is continually getting frustrated and agitated. She has gone and sat down next to some other patients but is still claiming she feels lost. John is asleep opposite me, sat at one of the dining room tables. Black and blue bruises are all over both his arms. He is wearing a bright blue polo shirt, but his face looks dull. Behind those closed eyes are years of experience, over 90 of them. Life experience that I cannot begin to explore. Maybe he still has snippets of his memory left, but today will not be a day we can try to discuss this. He has been asleep most of the day. Occasionally he stirs, and awakens, he stares intently at me with is deep brown eyes and moves both his hands towards me in an inquisitive manner. I try to understand what he is saying, but it just comes out as an awkward garbled mess of incoherent vowels and consonants. I reach out and touch his hand and he smiles, he taps my hands a few times, and then withdraws and quickly falls back asleep.

Elsie is sat next to me. She starts touching my feet, 'What size are you dear?' I reply I'm a 9. 'A 9 you say? Well you must be proud!'. She has long white hair, straggly with some faint curls at the ends; she wears a gold wedding ring around her neck and a purple cardigan.

Liz is on the move again. 'Nobody seems to be able to help me, 'D..I...F.'

Malcolm, who is now clutching an orange blanket, suddenly stumbles onto his feet. 'Right let's have this, I've got to get out of here', he shuffles past me and smiles. He walks into the lounge area and Iona barks at him 'Get OUT of here!' He carries on walking past her. There is an air of desperation in the air today, a real sense of false hope. A management plan needs to be formed. The current plan appears to be distraction, the phrase 'come and sit in your chair' has been used too many times to keep count, and it's just not having an impact any more, continually shifting people around like musical chairs. Everyone lost in a thick and murky fog, trying to claw their way out into the fresh crisp autumn air, to breathe that freshness once more, and get away from the stale hospital food smell that still lingers in the air.

John starts shouting 'PULL ME BACK! Gaffer'. There is an element of confusion. Does he want to be repositioned in his chair or be pulled back away from the table? I lower the chair for him and pull him away from the table. He seems to have calmed down now.

Elsie continues to stare intently at me, trying to burn holes in my head. She states that she is in love with me and wants to take me ballroom dancing sometime as soon as I am next available. She seems to be fretting about getting down to the village at some point today, she appears pleased that we both have the same colour eyes.

Liz is requesting help again; 'Nobody wants me.' She is now starting to push a wooden chair around the floor, using it as a makeshift walking frame, and she is in tears. A nurse and nursing assistant are helping to build an important looking jigsaw puzzle which is 300 pieces. Two other patients are also joining in on this task.

'Will you get my hands free and get the bloody lot of them,' John utters opposite me. 'Stop it!, bloody stop it Jarvis!'. He starts shaking uncontrollably, 'bloody stop it.'

'Where are you mom?' Liz shouts.

'Where are my stockings?' Elsie laughs out. I look through the window separating the dining room and lounge area. Iona is still in there watching TV, she shouts at me 'What's the matter then ?' looking perplexed.

Liz continues her impossible task. I glance at the clock, 4:15pm. It feels later than it is. 'It's almost time for dinner isn't it?' Elsie utters, she starts laughing again.

'Give me that card, bloody stop it, and bloody stop it, to get it...Bloody stop it'. John starts banging his hands on the table, still shaking, continuing to shout out, like a bizarre record that's stuck in its groove.

'Donald's girl did you say?' Elsie asks John. She begins laughing again, it is becoming a lot more of a menacing laugh by now.

By this point I'm wondering again why I went into mental health. I don't feel I can help these people to the best of my ability. It was apparently quite a common feeling, especially being this close to finishing. A lot of colleagues in my group were feeling the same way, we had talked about quitting the course numerous times, but I think all of us would regret it. At the end of the day, it was an important qualification to get, and once we had it, it could literally take you anywhere in the world. Australia, Canada, and New Zealand were all desperate for qualified nurses. These thoughts were always whirring away in the back of my mind, and in a way pushed me to carry on through it, and hopefully see the light at the end of the tunnel one day. Maybe I'm just upset as to the state of this hospital and how all the time it seems to come down to money and resources. I spoke to the activities co-ordinator the other day, and had a chat about what resources and things there were to do for the patients. She was quite honest and told me that all the activities budgets had been cut, so they were really feeling the pinch, and struggling to think of new and simple ideas that wouldn't cost much. The other day I had been so angry at the situation that I had frequented my local car boot sale and picked up half a dozen jigsaws for 50p each, and promptly bought them onto the ward for all the patients to use. The ward manager was very impressed at my thoughtfulness but then I shouldn't have to be buying the patients a few jigsaws. This hospital should have enough money and resources to fund these items themselves. It really does say something about how the place is run and what really is on offer for these patients. I realise not all the patients can make use of activities, unfortunately for some their dementia is too advanced for them to be able to contemplate or retain enough memory for even the simplest of tasks, but many of the other patients immediately took to doing some of the jigsaws that I had bought in for them, and at least it kept their attention for a few hours of the day. I often think to myself, it's no wonder that some patients get restless and agitated during the day, how would YOU feel if you were on a ward, day in, day out, with barely anything to keep you occupied throughout the day? I think I would soon be banging on those windows and trying the doors to get out very quickly indeed.

I glanced at my watch, it was coming up to 5pm. It should be time for a break around now. I had missed my lunch break due to the doctor's round. I secretly feel that Linda had planned this all along, again I just continued to grit my teeth and just think of the day when I would leave this establishment and no longer be a student. Breaks were often organised as follows: two members of staff would go from 12pm – 1pm, and another two would go from 1pm – 2pm. Afternoon breaks would normally be around 4.30pm – 5pm, and 5pm – 5.30pm. If you had a break at 5pm, this usually meant that you would miss most of tea time for the patients, and therefore not be required to help out with feeding, as often by the time you came back everyone had been fed and the food trolley was being packed away. I often didn't feel I needed the afternoon break, in some of my earlier placements I managed to get away with just having a half hour for lunch, and leaving the shift around 7pm instead of 8pm. I felt sometimes that the breaks just seemed to drag on, and it was a very long day until 8pm. How easy it was to get away would depend on the mentor you had. Some mentors were incredibly strict and by the book, so it wasn't always so easy.

At this moment in time Linda comes racing down the corridor straight in my direction. I groan silently to myself. She has that smile on her face again, I wonder what she can possibly want from me now.

Linda: Luveee, I think it's time you changed Stan's colostomy bag isn't it ?

'Err, yeah' I mutter, 'OK.'

Linda: I'll come with you, but you can do it, as you're a third year student, OK?

I follow Linda to the far end of the corridor.

Linda: Stan is already in his room, and I've got everything out ready for you, OK?

'Yeah, no problems.'

I walk into Stan's room. Stan hadn't been here very long. He was a very pleasant chap, and looked disturbingly like Alfie off Eastenders. Things hadn't been too good when he was first admitted here. Stan walked with a frame, and it took two members of staff to calm him down as he was swinging it wildly around trying to hit the walls and windows with it. Stan was in his mid 60s, and he had a few front teeth missing. He had short black greasy hair, and wore grey cardigans with green suit trousers. He was hoping to get discharged soon so he could live with his wife, who needed 24 hour care as she had lost both limbs in a car accident many years before. Stan had suffered from a nervous breakdown and couldn't cope with this situation any more, and was initially picked up by the police walking along the M6 motorway at 3am. Stan wasn't walking down the central reservation, he was walking *on* the M6. Luckily he was picked up quickly and admitted here for assessment.

Stan was sat on his bed, with his shirt unbuttoned and a smile on his face. Linda smiled and explained to Stan that I would be changing his bag, Stan agreed. I liked Stan. I would often get him up in the mornings and help get him washed and dressed, he would often have a good chat to me about what he used to do when he was younger, and his farm days of living on a large farm with his parents. This was part of the job you really relished, getting to know people from all different backgrounds and getting a little insight into what it was like for them growing up in totally different circumstances to your own.

I first had to clean around the stoma with some hot soapy water. This was the first time I had actually seen a stoma, and I was quite taken a-back. It really was just a hole that allowed the colostomy bag to attach to the large intestine. A stoma literally means 'mouth' in Greek. In this instance it was a surgically created opening which connected the large intestine to the outside environment, which then had a bag attached to it to allow the intestine to remove faeces out of the body, bypassing the rectum and drain into the pouch. I quickly cleaned around the area, and continued to talk to Stan whilst I was cleaning the area. I figured this was the best approach. Linda was breathing down my neck, probably relishing every moment and just waiting for me to look disgusted or comment, but I was too professional for that. I had done worse things during my training, and I was not to be beaten. I had a fresh colostomy bag to attach. It was surprisingly easy actually, and Stan didn't appear to be in any discomfort. Only when carefully removing the old bag did Stan wince just a little bit. I had some spray to use around the area to make the removal that little bit easier, but there were just a few places where it tugged just a little. On the whole though it was a very successful job, and more importantly, I had proved to Linda that I could do it, and would not be ground down by her inane cheerfulness. I cleaned up, buttoned Stan's shirt back up for him, and made my way back towards the lounge area. It was time for a break. Andrew was also due for a break too. We never really spoke outside of the ward, as he would just sleep in his car during his break time. He needed some 'down time'. I confess there have been times where I have gone for a quick power nap during lunch time. The quickest nap I had was about 10 minutes. Just enough to charge you up for the remainder of the shift. You never knew how good a shift you were going to have until you started it really, and from what I have found, it was all about the staff you worked with, not the patients. A really good team of staff who could joke around but also be hard working and professional really made the day go quickly and easily.

Andrew strolled out of the cloakroom, and came up towards me. 'See you in half an hour my good friend'.

'Yeah, no worries' I utter. Andrew really was a genuine 'good guy'. He never faltered, even after today's shift, he still had all the energy to motivate himself and most importantly still carried that smile on his face. I exit the ward and walk over to my car. It was a cold and windy evening, and it was already dark, which made me feel quite depressed. There was no one about, and the leaves gently rustled along by the abandoned church nearby. I looked up at the ward building, into the small windows which were just pitch black. This really was quite a creepy place. I made a mental note to myself not to work here when I qualified as a nurse. This wasn't the area for me. Not by a long way.

5pm – 7:45pm

Having made a few phone calls and texted a few people, it was time to enter back into the ward for the final leg of the shift. Andrew was just getting out of his car and so we walked into the ward together. Tea time would be about half way through by now.

'Looking forward to going home soon hey?', Andrew comments. 'Yeah, I sure am' I respond. Today had been quite a long day, every day was to be honest. Most days were fairly routine, but with mental health you never knew what was around the corner. It could all change so quickly and so dramatically. As we walked back onto the ward, the sounds of clinking plates were still to be heard. Tea was probably just about to finish. Once I had left the cloakroom, I walked back into the lounge area and asked if I could help with anything. Linda was busy doing the tea time drugs. She never included me in the drugs rounds, but I didn't mind. The least time I spent with her the better really. She wasn't my mentor anyway, and so it didn't really matter too much about spending a great deal of time with her. Your mentor was supposed to guide you through each placement, helping you with any areas that you were unsure about, and observing how you dealt with certain areas of nursing, such as personal care, moving and handling, infection control, etc., etc. As you progressed through your training, each placement area had various forms and tick boxes that had to be signed off and completed in order to prove your competence in each area. Usually every third placement would involve an even thicker document in which you had many more competencies to pass and be signed off by a qualified mentor. At first they seemed very difficult, but you got used to them as you progressed through your training. You often got the impression that many mentors found the process a real pain, and were soon quick to sign off your documents so that you wouldn't need to bother them so much. I could see their point in one respect. They didn't get any extra money for being a mentor, but then they had to bear the increase in workload on top of their normal nursing duties. In some cases the NHS trust would send the nurses on mentorship training as a requirement, whether they liked to be a mentor or not. This was bad practice. It started to mean that the nurses only way of improving their pay band was to do a mentorship course. Not because they wanted to do it, but just because this was the only way to essentially further their career.

Valencia and the student nurse were busying themselves picking up plates and various cutlery, and tidying up. Most of the patients were sat in the lounge. Iona was sat in the other room in her own chair. She had seen me, and was waving me over to her. Iona said what she thought, and was very direct in her thinking. A lot of the other patients riled her, and she liked things her own particular way. I got on with her usually, but you certainly had to be on the ball and pay attention to her, or she would have no problems in tearing strips off you verbally. She had light greying hair, and quite a elongated face, with piercing green eyes, which would watch your every move, staring at you continually. Her voice was that of an old schoolteacher, and she spoke loudly all the time. She would often be moved into the other room just to let the other patients get some peace as like earlier today she could quite happily start shouting at any of them and her words were often fairly unkind. Iona wasn't as vocal as she could be though, she had recently had her dose of Haloperidol increased, and this had seemed to have a dramatic effect on her mood at times. Haloperidol was an older form of antipsychotic medication. Antipsychotics were used a lot in Dementia, even though they weren't licensed for that particular use. They were used to help control people's agitation and aggression, but like all drugs could have particular side effects, the most common and controversial one being tardive dyskenisia which can be involuntary muscular movements, primarily of the face, jaw, arms or legs. Antipsychotics were often coming under some pressure due to these side effects and the fact that maybe we were using them as a 'chemical cosh' in order to subdue and stop our patients from moving and making them too tired to do anything. Iona looked very pale and frightened as she spoke to me.

'Love, don't take it away from me, I know what they have done to me you know, I feel awful, I cannot move, I'm telling you now there is something going on here.'

'It's OK Iona, you're safe here, we are here to look after you', I say calmly. Iona was often a little paranoid, but I hadn't seen her looking this worried for a long time.

'Hold my hand would you love'. Iona talked in quite a thick East London accent. She had spent a long time living there as a seamstress, until eventually her health deteriorated and she went back to live with her daughter in Wolverhampton. She had been diagnosed with Dementia in 2005, and was now in the end stages. Her daughter had found it too difficult to cope and moved Iona into a nursing home. The nursing home could not cope with Iona's behaviour and verbal and sometimes physical aggression, which is why she currently came to be here at the hospital. I heard the other day that the home is willing to have her back now since she has been assessed here and we have 'improved' her mental state. This has been improved through increases of her medication, primarily Haloperidol.

I outstretch my hand and hold Iona's hand. She smiles at me, and her face immediately softens and warms. I almost forget the rage and violent nature of her verbal outbursts from before. Iona is clearly scared and has some degree of possible insight. She knows something has changed.

'Love, just hold me hand will you, I will appreciate it, you can't trust anyone round here I tell you, all complete wankers if you ask me, don't let them see the whites of your eyes son, or you could be next. Fuckers, the lot of them.'

'It's OK Iona' I assure her. 'I'm here, and I will keep my eyes open don't you worry'.

'I know you will lad, I know, you're the smart one, I know, I'm not stupid you know, what's your name again?'

'Jack.'

Iona laughs. 'Jack', that's it, that's my boy, training to be a doctor aren't you, well you keep at it, you do your paperwork and you will be fine, and be a doll, keep looking after people like me, because I won't be around forever you know'.

'I'll keep it up don't you worry, I'm training to be a nurse though' I smile.

'Nurse, doctor, I don't fucking know, you carry on son anyway, leave me here, but do me a favour first won't you ? Put me in front of the telly won't you, I want to watch the telly now, see what's on, but put the volume up loud, me ears aren't what they used to be you know, deaf as a fucking post lately.'

I let go of Iona's hand, and slowly push her chair around so she is facing the television in the corner. I turn the volume up loud.

'How is that?' I ask.

'Perfect, now come here so I can speak to you properly.'

I crouch and sit in front of Iona. She leans down to me and whispers in my ear. 'Be a good lad, I don't think I've got long left in this world you know, I feel awful, something is definitely wrong here, I know it's wrong, they have done something to me, they have, I'm not stupid, I know it's wrong, you go and tell them, and I will be safe then.'

'It's OK Iona, I'll let them know' I whisper.

Iona smiles at me, pats my hand with hers. She leans in further to speak into my ear.

'Do me a favour now and fuck off love. I want to watch the telly in peace.'

I glance at my watch. It was getting on for 7pm. The shift had almost come to an end. It had been a fairly average day, although there was never one day the same in mental health. It was a very physically and mentally demanding role, and it was one I was certainly thinking a lot about, and thinking where I would be in the future. At this time of the day everything was pretty much done. Linda had finished the tea time medication, and had buried herself in the office with a mountain of paperwork. Andrew was sat down in the lounge area watching a Britain's funniest home movies show on the television. He still didn't look fazed. There were a few patients walking up and down the corridor, a little restless, but mainly everyone was sat either in the lounge area and sleeping. I had realised I still hadn't opened the envelope I had got this morning in the post. It was still in my rucksack. As it was a quiet moment I decided to go and get my backpack and get the envelope out. As it was so close to my training nearing completion I had already begun to apply for some jobs. Sadly there were not a great deal of opportunities open initially. Most jobs were still within the elderly sector, and in terms of hospital jobs, they were only offering six month temporary contracts. I had already made my mind up about working in a hospital environment. I wasn't going to do it. I felt that the hospitals were not offering enough for the patients here, and often the morale of the staff and the lack of staff made a severe impact on how we were then able to spend time with the patients. We learnt at university all the time about patient led care, and often we were simply too busy with all the paperwork and bureaucracy of the establishment to give enough of our time to them.

I had actually applied for three jobs, one of which was going to be a private nursing home with two separate dementia units. I was hoping that the envelope would be some good news from at least one of these applications I had sent off a few weeks ago. I go to get my rucksack and pull out the envelope in my bag, quickly opening it.

As I opened up the letter, it was indeed from the private nursing home I had applied to. It was a letter asking me to attend an interview. A smile broke out on my face. At last an opportunity for a job! I stuff the letter back in my rucksack, and walk back down the corridor and towards Andrew.

'Hey, how's it going ?' I utter.

'Not too bad my friend' Andrew smiles.

'Guess what!, I've got a job interview at a private nursing home!' I exclaim to Andrew

'Great news my friend, you will be a good nurse, you are a very hard working person my friend' Andrew replies.

I sure hope I would be. Having been through so much already, I was really wondering what it would be like to become a real mental health nurse. I glance back at Linda in the office, still writing away, and start to think to myself, do I really want this? Can I become that person, or I can I craft my own way of doing things and be my own nurse, and rise above all this bureaucracy ?

There was not much to do now except wait until the clock struck 7.45pm. Linda never let me go early, not once. I was lucky enough this evening that she had some extra paperwork to be getting on with that she couldn't pass on to me. It wouldn't be much longer now anyway. I glance at some of the patients. Iona is sleeping in her chair now. Liz has calmed down a lot more and is smiling at me from a chair she is sat down on. I feel so sorry for these patients, but I have to hope that my skills as a student can start helping these people in the future, and that we can challenge the system and its financial motivations and really start getting back to basics, and start thinking about the person, and their perspective of their illness. It really isn't rocket science, and that is why I came into Mental Health in the first place; because I wanted to help people. Their lived experiences. Their stories. This is what life is about, and only when you have spoken to people and their relatives can you begin to start discovering who that person is and the experiences they have been through. I glance up at the clock; it's 7.40pm. Andrew is now standing up and walking towards me. It is time to go and get our coats. The night staff have just come through the green door. A nurse and a carer. Fresh and ready for another 12 hour night shift.

I walk into the cloakroom with Andrew and get my coat and rucksack. We exit out of the cloakroom, and then hover outside the office, where Linda is now finalising her paperwork and the night staff are tucking into a few biscuits and cup of tea in the office.

Myself and Andrew look up at the clock. It's 7.45pm. Linda looks at me and smiles that smile she has been giving me all day and says 'OK you can go now luvee, see you bright and early tomorrow'.

'Yeah'. I reply. I sure will. But not for much longer, I think.

I walk out of the green doors with Andrew. Andrew turns to me.

'You're done my friend. The shift is over, see you tomorrow'.

Mental Health

I glance up at the pitch black sky, a full moon illuminating the car park. I wonder to myself what the future will hold as I make my way towards my car. Another shift closer to my eventual career.

Voluntary Services – A diary of events

At the start of my second year of training, it was required of us to arrange for our own placement area, as long as it was connected to the voluntary services, which could incorporate a large area of organisations, even including charity shops! In order to get a rounded experience I decided to pick two different areas to compare and contrast, one being with a local charity, but also one which was well known throughout the country. The other was independent and provided a short drop in centre for people with mental health issues, generally older people, but there would still be quite a large range of people who were in the younger age brackets. The following is a complete diary of events covering the twelve weeks of placement time spent within the two organisations.

If I'm considering reading a diary, I would always think about taking it off the shelf or whatever coffee table it is lying on, (having asked permission of whoever's diary it was) and read the first paragraph (although I guess most diaries don't have paragraphs, I guess it depends?) If no one was around, and I couldn't find the owner of the diary, then I would probably quickly sneak a look at it anyway (I know, I'm a bad person, but curiosity is a killer).

I think the first paragraph to a diary or book is a good indicator of whether or not you are going to like what's ahead, so imagine the pressure I'm under now to please you, the reader, I'm not sure exactly how many people are going to read this diary, and if it's just myself, then in effect I'm talking to myself, which could be considered the first sign of madness although if you're talking to yourself through the written word, is that the same as actually talking to out loud to yourself?

Basically this is a diary of events, which originally did start out to be a very small diary, but I think as my experiences have grown, I think I have managed to grow the size of the diary into a near monolithic proportion. You might be wondering how I know the diary is so big, when this is only the introduction to it, well you have caught me red handed. You see the beauty of information technology is that I can edit beginnings, middle and ends whenever I like, add new bits here and there, and basically change the whole structure around, but you're spoiling the illusion, just treat it as the beginning, and take it from there.

I hope this diary will not be too boring for people. I am going to try and make it as interesting as possible, this diary is not promising to be a laugh a minute read, or indeed a serious tome, but merely a reflection of events covering my voluntary placement experiences. Often I will be writing in the first person, but sometimes switch to third person. I hope this does not offend anyone, but it's just my way of writing, and I may even include some tales that I find amusing or anecdotes along the way. I will say now, and this will probably be quite obvious, that I'm no writer, so do excuse any grammatical areas that may crop uP, remember **NO onE Is Perfecttt.**

If you're still with me, then I would consider this diary sold. If I've managed to hook your interest from this brief introduction then I consider you interested in what I have to say. I like diaries with short little sections, and diaries which offer a considerable amount of emotions and feelings that people have at the time, not that I've read many diaries, but of the ones I have begged to read, I think the best ones are the ones that people really put their heart into. I can tell you now, this diary is not going to be like: 'day 23, went to meet friends, had a coffee, went home' style of writing, and indeed you may get fed up with my somewhat long prose at times, but hey, you wanted to read this diary right? So I figure you should read it to the end, to get a full picture and maybe more of an insight into me and my experiences.

I shall bore you no more, and shall start with the very first day, of the very first placement! Enjoy, and see you at the end...

Your friend in time...

Jack

8/1

<u>Breedan</u>: **'Ain't a hard time been invented that I cannot handle.'**

(Heat, 1995)

I went and met the other two students who I would be working with at Voluntary (to protect confidentiality of the voluntary placement, each placement will be referred to as 'Voluntary'). We were all told to meet up at 1.30pm. I wasn't sure what to expect from the meeting, and presumably it would be to discuss what we would be doing at Voluntary. When I got there we were met by one of the main workers there and she had prepared a large list of events and activities she thought we could get involved with. She was very keen on us being able to spread the word about Voluntary and what they were about, including going to schools and colleges and presenting information about them.

This idea initially filled me with dread. I had foolishly thought that working within the voluntary sector would mean that I wouldn't have to replicate similar skills and activities that we had already done at University many times over! Presentations were not my favourite of activities; so to say I'm feeling anxious now is an understatement.

Many of the other activities sounded much more interesting. She suggested fund raising ideas such as a car boot sale, and maybe getting the service users involved in some sort of cooking event and teaching them about healthy eating. These things were much more to my liking, and we eventually decided on doing a car boot sale for fund raising, organising a healthy eating lunch, and investigating areas where we could do some presentations, including local colleges. I couldn't believe it! **CAR BOOT SALES!** I'd only spent half my life going round car boot sales, I knew the areas, I knew the score, and this was something I would be able to do quite confidently!

The rest of the afternoon was spent gathering phone numbers for local schools and colleges; I felt that my colleagues were a bit too eager to ring around lots of colleges before even considering what we would actually be presenting! I had come to Voluntary to find out what they were about, and here we were talking about presenting our knowledge, before even I knew what I was talking about! I did not voice my concerns about this as I thought it would seem like I didn't want to be bothered to work, and this was not the case. I was just a bit anxious about lining up too many areas and not being prepared.

As first days go, this was quite a stressful one for me! After my colleague had rung around a few places, we decided to go to the pub (for a serious discussion of course, it's not all about the beers!). I began to give a few ideas on how I thought we should do a presentation, and how we should do a PowerPoint for it, which I was comfortable with.

After our meeting I still felt anxious and a little worried as to whether I had picked the right sort of placement! I found it strange that we had not met a single service user and here we were being expected to organise all these different events without having spoken to anyone who actually uses the service. I would have thought it best to discuss various groups and ideas with the people who actually use the service and get their ideas first hand. I felt it a little rushed and felt that we were left to our own devices a bit too much. I understood that we were to be more self directed and take more responsibility for our learning, but this felt like quite a large step and a very quick one at that!

9/1

<u>Lt. Col. Frank Slade</u>**:** **[***shouting***]** **I'm in the dark, here!**

(Scent of a Woman, 1992)

I was meeting today with another colleague of mine at my second voluntary placement. I had worked there before for a day, so knew what to expect. I was told that the main person in charge wanted to speak to us together at 9.30am. I assumed it would be just for a quick chat and to sort out what hours he wanted each of us to work. When I got there it was quite apparent that he was expecting us to be there for most of the day. Initially I was quite annoyed about this, as I was not anticipating being there for the whole day, which to some extent was my own fault as I could have checked with him if I had really wanted to find out why he wanted to see us, but I found I soon settled back in and some of the people recognised me from before so I was able to strike up a rapport again with some familiar faces.

I still felt a bit on edge as the placement is quite relaxed and laid back, there is no set structure and a lot of the people who use the service are quite old, so they cannot be involved in any major physical activities, there is not even a television there, although there is a pool table, and I figure that this could be a good opportunity for me to build more friendships with the users.

My colleague and I were left to our own devices, we felt a bit left out, most people were talking to themselves, I don't mean actually talking to themselves, I mean talking with other people, and I guess what I mean then is AMONGST themselves.

The major problem I have sometimes with a place like this is that you don't want to be too intrusive. Whilst you are there to help people and get on with them, I sometimes feel a bit of an outsider and feel it strange to just suddenly sit next to people and start chatting. A lot of people simply don't like strangers coming up to them and talking, so I was initially a bit wary of trying to force myself upon people, and it was clear a lot of people were a bit paranoid towards me as they kept staring at me, which unnerved me considerably.

I decided to talk to people, who started talking to me, and I would progress as the weeks went by. I thought this was the best strategy, and it seemed to work well. I thought there was no point trying to be the expert student nurse (well, technically 'volunteer') and going in guns blazing talking to everyone and trying to be liked, it simply wasn't going to happen that way, play it cool I thought, let friendships build! I agreed with the boss that I would be coming to this placement only on a Wednesday due to my other commitments, and he was fine with that. I felt pleased now that I had got two placements.

10/11

<u>Nicholas</u>: **Did I have a choice? Did I have a choice?**

(The Game, 1997)

I was back at Voluntary, still anxious about the presentation side of things, although I began to feel more at home with my colleagues as we were all in the same boat, and as we had agreed to do the presentations together, I did start to feel a bit better. I do think it's a strange thing to ask someone to 'promote' something when they don't actually know anything about the 'product' initially, I think I finally figured that it was going to happen no matter what, so I should stop trying to worry so much about it, and start being more professional, and see it like a job, or an assignment, and try to spin it in a more positive light. At the end of the day, I thought, I'm bound to have to do more University presentations in the next few years, so doing presentations might improve my confidence more.

We had got two meetings set up today. One was with a local workshop. They wanted to meet with us about our idea to present to their workers about Voluntary. The meeting went well and they seemed very nice, they said we would be presenting in the canteen! A very small canteen too! I suddenly realised the reality kicking in; we were actually going to do this, and a date was set for the 28th February. They said they would also help us with making a poster for our car boot sale.

After the meeting we then popped into a women's institute, as I had managed to make contact the night before, and they said they had a kitchen we could use for our lunch idea. The kitchen was a good size, but there were no eating facilities, and the kitchen was down long winding steps which was going to be tricky for access. They suggested going to a local hall. We went there in the pouring rain only to find that it was shut. My colleague rang them up, and they said we would have to pop by next week and come and inspect the premises.

The next meeting wasn't till 2pm, at the Sixth Form College, quite a big gap, so my colleague and I went our separate ways for a bit (our other colleague was going to meet us later as she wasn't with us for our morning meetings).

Walking into the Sixth Form was a bit daunting, for no other reason that I could explain except that it was full of teenagers, hardly surprising really! But for some reason I seem to feel self conscious when lots of teenagers are about, probably due to me having a milestone birthday this year of 30! Maybe I just feel too old now!

Anyway we sat down with one of the main teachers responsible for health and social care, and we pitched our presentation (I don't know how we managed this as we hadn't actually got one yet!) She thought it would be best if we set up a stand where students could come to us and ask us about Voluntary, rather than a talk. I breathed a massive sigh of relief (internally!) Thank god for that!

That was it for the day, success; people want us to spread the word. Fantastic.

15/1

Just feel like shooting something today!

Meeting today at Voluntary with my other student colleagues, packed my laptop, confident of a proper brainstorming session. I had spent all night working on a PowerPoint presentation and some poster ideas so we could develop further.

Once we got there we met up with some staff at Voluntary, and explained our progress so far, met one of the managers there, and he said that we could use his PowerPoint to help us do our presentations for Voluntary. Well that didn't exactly cheer me up! I'd worked most of the night on my own! After that we didn't seem to have anything else to discuss, I showed my poster ideas, the other colleagues said that was fine, I felt a little underwhelmed and was unsure what I was doing there to be honest, I'd worked hard all night, and this meeting didn't seem to have any agenda at all, maybe it was my own fault for not raising issues, but I felt like I'd done my bit the night before, and that we should just be working on more things, however it just seemed to be a discussion about general University work. My other colleague shared the same reservations, and said she didn't understand why were doing all this extra work on top of our University work, we had thought we were just going to be getting involved in groups with service users and getting to know them.

I don't understand how we can develop our experiences by just promoting Voluntary with presentations, I don't feel like we're with the actual people that matter, maybe things will improve, I just feel a little disappointed with how it's working at the minute. I'm used to self directed work, but this doesn't seem to have any structure at all. The staff today at Voluntary didn't seem helpful either, we weren't getting any feedback really, it's almost like we have been sidelined as 'students' and just left to it, and as long as we spread the word about them and what they do, and raise a bit of money then it will be fine, to me that does not feel quite correct.

Hopefully things will improve, but today felt like a huge waste of my time, nothing new was gained, we just made a poster for our stand, and it felt like everyone was just very unhelpful.

16/1

<u>Catherine</u>: **Killing isn't like smoking. You can stop.**

(Basic Instinct, 1992)

Back to listen and care today. My other student colleague was told that she needed to speak to more people, and not just the same people. We had a discussion on how it wasn't always appropriate to go up to people and speak to them. I didn't see that it was necessary to be bothering people all of the time. I decided to go up to a few people today, but not force myself upon people, I said hello to a lot of the regulars, a lot recognised me, but I still felt a bit on edge and a bit awkward. Maybe I just need to get more used to the environment, or maybe I don't feel like I've enough experience of this sort of environment yet.

The difficulty sometimes is that there are mainly older people who use the centre, and so there is a large age gap between us. Some of the older women seem to ignore me, I'm not sure if this is because of their mental health, or just simply that they don't think that they can relate anything with me or have anything in common. Maybe I'm being a bit paranoid about it.

I did meet a nice gentleman who told me all about how he had his hip replaced, and that he came to the centre most days for a bit of company. He engaged well with me, and I felt quite pleased that I had got some rapport going with him. At times I feel a bit pressured to go and speak to people, but this conversation seemed to happen quite naturally.

My big concern at the moment is that the manager of the centre wants to try and help promote healthy eating to the group, but still continues to stock fizzy drinks and crisps for the users to purchase. I'm also not happy that one of the users brings his daughter in on the odd days and continues to feed her biscuits and jam sandwiches. The user himself is very obese, so I don't agree with the example he is setting for his child.

I don't feel comfortable in trying to address these healthy eating issues yet, but I think that there needs to be more information and education going on as regards healthy eating. At least if there was a choice of healthier options people would be able to make a decision, but it seems extremely limited. I'm wondering if should mention this to the manager in the weeks to come, and maybe try and push a healthier approach. I don't think it's my place to speak to the service user about his daughter, I feel I might alienate part of the group if I try get on a moral high ground! Although at the same time I'm thinking maybe it's just a lack of education about healthier options, I think I will try and slowly mention about healthier options to the manager and see if we can implement some sort of change. All in all quite an interesting day, I even got to sit in on a forum meeting where the users were able to discuss some issues that they were concerned about. It was good to see that they could voice opinions to people outside the service and try to initiate changes where possible.

17/1

<u>Austin Powers</u>: **Yeah, baby, yeah**

(Austin Powers, 1997)

Had to go to the hall today to meet the owner, with regards to seeing its suitability for our healthy eating lunch for the service users of Voluntary. Supposed to be meeting my other student colleague there, but she couldn't make it, she had overslept! It was going to be all down to me! The meeting went well, he was a very nice man, I had to shout quite loud in his right ear as he was quite deaf, and the sounds of my dulcet tones reverberated around the huge hall in a strange sort of echo.

He showed me around the hall, which was huge, and had plenty of good kitchen facilities. In fact it was perfect, my only worry now is how we are going to get people interested and attending! It's going to be quite a challenge, but we have a few weeks to start arranging who might be interested.

I felt a bit better after this. Something positive had happened at least, but I still feel at a bit of a loss as to our real purpose with Voluntary, maybe it will start coming together in the next few weeks, let's hope so. Went home straight afterwards. My other student colleague suggested I should drop in to Voluntary and meet the service users to mention about the lunch idea and put it to them. I didn't feel comfortable in doing this on my own, I had spent an hour at the hall, and didn't feel it was fair that I should be running around doing everything on my own, plus I think I was a bit anxious speaking to a group, I think it's going to be better if we all go together. I'm going to suggest this to the other members of my group, and hopefully sort this out for next week.

Whilst at home I began to work on the PowerPoint for our presentation. I'm doing most of the computer work at the minute, but I'm happy to be doing that as I'm quite comfortable with technical things.

I think I need to suggest to my other colleague to take on more work if she can as she only has one placement so it will be harder for her to make up her hours, whereas myself and the other colleague have another placement to go to, so it's also unfair for us to be doing the same level of work. I think we need a proper meeting next week and I should raise these points.

22/1

<u>Jack Torrance</u>: **HERE'S JOHNNY.**

(The Shining, 1980)

AAAGHHHHH! I'm feeling stressed. I don't normally suffer from stress, but I feel a bit stressed today. I went to the local psychiatric hospital canteen for a meeting with the rest of my colleagues, again to discuss what we were doing for Voluntary. We had a PowerPoint ready, but I stressed that we needed to see the actual service users and discuss with them what they would like to do! I find the whole process very confusing, it could turn out that we have been doing all this work for nothing. Setting up a place for the cooking at the hall could all be a big waste of time. It turns out that they rang back to say we couldn't have our original date, which was quite handy as we were in University on that date anyway! (as I had ballsed up the dates on my calendar.) I think it could work, but again we all discussed how we weren't being supported in our placement, and decided to take things into our own hands and go meet one of the groups on Monday after University so at least we can get to meet some service users. After the meeting, I came home to an email from the training director at Voluntary saying that I needed to complete their core training before working with any of their service users. One of the days falls on a University day! I'm getting frustrated! I need to maybe take out frustrations on a computer game.

I do not want to miss University, so I contact the University and it turns out that I can do the training, but need to see the lecturer about the session I'm going to miss. This is all going a bit wrong, it seems like nothing but meetings and no action, at least we are going in on Monday to go and meet some service users! I was told that Voluntary's training is very similar to what we already have done at University. I'm feeling a bit annoyed today, I can't decide if it's the weather or just how generally shit things are going with the placement, maybe things will improve, I'll have to wait until Monday, but at the moment I just feel like we are being used as cheap labour to promote Voluntary, and I still feel uncomfortable in doing this as I'm not entirely sure what the organisation does yet! This is not progressing my learning!

Just received a phone call from Voluntary, saying how they want to speak to us next week! Well, I said we were coming in on Monday anyway so they could meet us then, I hope this will finally offer some support that we need, we have done as much as we can in our limited capacity, I think it's time to sit down and get some help, I will remain optimistic! I'll try and relax now and not think about it till next week, to have a bit of focus would be nice!!

23/1

Other placement today, I felt more part of the team today, I was asked to help one of the service users to go and get his breakfast from the local café, he had recently undergone an operation on his throat, and was a bit unsteady on his legs. I got on well with him and we seemed to have quite a bit in common, even though he was 73 years of age, we discussed the benefits of juicing, and he was very keen on telling me all about his past and about his family. I was making progress, and I felt like I was actually doing some good at last. When we had finished breakfast we went back to listen and care and continued to chat. I made him a cup of tea, but not long afterwards he suddenly got up out of his chair and rushed towards the exit. I didn't know why he had done this, I went and followed him to check if he was OK, but he was throwing up in the toilet, all I could sheepishly ask him if he was OK, which he clearly wasn't! I asked him if he wanted a glass of water but he declined. I managed to encourage him to go outside and have some fresh air, he seemed quite humbled by the gesture, he said he had eaten too much breakfast, he had only got out of hospital the previous day, and only just been able to eat solid foods again, so I think his breakfast was a bit too much for him and put his system into a bit of shock. I stayed with him until his son picked him up; he wished me all the best and said he would probably see me next week.

I felt very sorry for him, but also considered that at least I was there for him to talk to. It might have been a bit embarrassing for him, but maybe I helped take the edge of this.

What I noticed today more than anything was how the regular users of the centre seemed very ill. I don't know if this is me becoming more aware of mental health, and a combination of me recognising how these users normally act, but there was definitely a sliding slope of illness. The one chap I spoke to didn't recognise me at first and was incredibly paranoid, he did apologise for this, but he wasn't his normal self. I spoke to another young man who seemed obsessed with everything being his fault, he thought the police were going to shoot him, and stated that he had even rung up the police himself and they said that he hadn't done anything wrong. I tried to assure him that everything was fine but he just didn't seem to listen.

I sometimes feel I am patronising people by saying things will be OK, how do I know this? It's also a difficult thing to try and convey genuinely, there were definitely some very ill people here today! An older lady kept running up to me and seemed to have increasingly delusional thoughts and pressure of speech (this is a tendency to speak rapidly and frenziedly). I couldn't even understand what she was saying at one point but she kept talking about a thousand words per minute, and I wasn't quite sure what to do except just nod at key moments!! I felt quite sad during the afternoon, it's like I'm in a film of my own creation and everyone here are the characters in my story, as I look from right to left I see people's faces looking at me, almost like they want answers from me, but I can't seem to help them. I'm questioning my role in this group and feel out of my depth sometimes, however I think I am also beginning to realise how much of a help this group is to people, this is really all some people have got!

At one point it was all getting to me quite a lot, and I really started feeling like I'd taken on too much, how on earth am I going to continue with this course?! Maybe these doubts are normal, maybe these kinds of experiences are going to shape me as a professional, sometimes I seem to distance myself and I do feel trapped in my own film like a recreation of life, spinning around uncontrollably, people talking and shouting, how can I help them? It's almost dreamlike.

I feel so guilty when I go home, almost humbled as I step into my living room and see the piles of multimedia devices and media formats designed to distract me from my everyday life, and think how lucky I actually am. I think today has started to really define me and my role within mental health, these people need support and they need the interaction, to some that is their only life line, and it's starting to fit more clearly now, I only hope I can develop now and provide these people with a bit of interaction. Some of the people who weren't speaking to me last week came over and spoke to me, I think I'm starting to let my own paranoia and insecurities cloud my judgement at times, some of these people simply don't have the confidence to speak to me or feel intimidated by a new volunteer, I must respect this and do my best to help these people in whatever way I can.

Today has made me look at my life slightly differently. I'm beginning to appreciate my own life a little more; when I speak to people at the group I realise some of the hardships that some people have gone through, and for some they are making a huge effort to simply get up in the mornings and come to this centre in which they feel valued and can interact with their friends.

I'm still no closer on trying to introduce healthier foods to the group or suggest it to the manager. I didn't think it was appropriate today; it seemed to ground me a little more in reality, and I think I have finally begun to see how people's moods can alter one week to the next, something I didn't quite grasp on my other placements. Maybe I am becoming more experienced but not always realising it, maybe the more I speak and interact, the more my knowledge will grow and shape me as an individual. One thing is for sure though; I definitely need to play a game of pool with someone there next week! I don't think I can handle just sitting down all the time!

28/1

Today was a University day, but we had decided to go to the drop in group after our lecture. It ran from 1pm – 3pm, and we thought it would be a good chance to finally meet some service users! When we got there, there were a few volunteers from Voluntary, and a few service users. We had a brief introduction, and discussed some of our ideas with Voluntary about the cooking and fund raising ideas we had. We had already discussed these before, but they just wanted to see how we were getting on so far. Well, we had to explain that everything was set up, but we just needed service users' opinions! We decided to put a notice up on the whiteboard in the main lounge about the cooking and lunch idea, and stated that people could put their names down for it so we could start getting an idea for numbers. Initially the service users were quite reserved, but once we started talking about it more, a few started to put their names down.

I felt more comfortable today. It was initially daunting meeting new service users, but then I've found it always has been, no matter what placement I've been on, however the main difference here is that it felt like a step in the right direction, and some of the people there were very nice, we even managed to have a game of hangman with a new service user who seemed initially quite reserved, but she seemed to enjoy herself in our company.

One of the chaps there came up to me and asked were we going to visit the groups often, I said we would try to visit more but we couldn't promise what days or when due to our time constraints with our other projects. Immediately afterwards a volunteer came up to me and told me to avoid speaking to this service user and to give him space. I felt a bit nervous after this, and then proceeded to watch this service user sit down and have a good chat with the rest of the service users and one of my student colleagues. I thought that was a bit strange, maybe he didn't like men, or maybe he just didn't like students, oh well, at least I was told. I assume he may have some sort of issue so best not to question the volunteer's word. I also passed this information on to the other student colleague, all in all I felt happy today, initially nervous, but glad I came, and we seemed to get along with at least one service user and engage her in some games and chat.

We also managed to get some display boards and posters today for our stand at the Sixth Form, and hopefully the University.

The size of the bag seemed to resemble an ocean, which gave everyone a good laugh as I tried to teeter down the stairs with it on my shoulder, and then put it in the boot of my car like some oversized red holdall designed for dead bodies. It looks like I've taken half of the Voluntary organisation with me and discreetly popped it all in my boot. Ah well, it's all good fun.

29/1

I had a meeting today with my other student colleagues, to talk about our presentation. To date we still only have one presentation. I'm silently happy about this, inside my head I'm jumping for joy! Well, I understand the importance of presentations but I feel it's a little too eager to try and set ourselves up with too much work, I mean there's already enough work to satisfy a small country for about 3 years, and this is only the START of the second year! I'm kind of feeling that maybe one or two presentations would be sufficient; I had a nightmare the other day that we had set up about twelve presentations and it was just awful, luckily in reality, at the moment, we have one presentation, and two hours of managing a stand for Voluntary at the Sixth Form College and possibly one day at the University. I also spoke to a friend of mine who might be able to get us a presentation at another college, he's a psychology teacher so he might be able to pull those strings of power and get us in to present to his class. Whether that will happen or not I'm not sure, but at least it's a good contact, and some good might come of it.

We decided today to work out what we were actually going to say in our presentation. As one of our colleagues already did some befriending, we thought it best she talked about her own experiences of this. I was going to concentrate more on the types of groups that Voluntary offered, at least I could talk about the Monday chat group confidently, now I had actually attended it! I don't think it's going to be too bad really; I'm more worried now about making the presentation seem interesting and exciting for people, and if we as a group don't find it interesting then our core audience certainly isn't going to! The main way to combat this I feel is going to be through pictures. Of course we have to be careful here in case we want to show pictures of the chat groups and the people involved, because if we include service users in pictures, then of course there could be some conflict of interest and confidentiality issues unless we gain their consent first.

At least we had decided what sort of areas to discuss, as the presentation was at the workshop, and in their canteen we couldn't be relying on a power point this time so we thought it best to create some cue cards to help us vocalise what we were going to talk about. At this point I don't see how our presentation is going to last that long, certainly not half an hour anyway! Still at least we seem more organised now in our structure and have decided on a loose subject area.

My mood feels OK today, again I feel that some of the areas we have discussed are tying together a bit more and making more sense. I'm still not happy with the lack of support we are getting from our 'support worker' at Voluntary, and she's leaving in two weeks! I just feel we could be more included in things; OK, we went to the chat group on a Monday, but that was our decision, no one is telling us what to do, which in one way can be quite liberating, and we are able to control and organise our days accordingly, but on the other hand, I think it would be nice to have some support now and again, especially as I've had no experience of a voluntary placement such as this! Still things might get better after next week, because we are doing our voluntary training, although the organiser of the training said we need to bring our CRB checks along. I'm thinking that mine has expired by now, so I hope they don't want us to go and get another new one, that will cause all sorts of complications again! Oh well, see what happens.

30/1

Another placement day; it turns out that the lady who was talking to me last week with pressure of speech and clearly delusional thought has been admitted to the local psychiatric hospital, now whilst this is clearly quite upsetting for her (I can only imagine, given the circumstances that I heard) in some ways I feel that this is the best place for her, judging from how she appeared to me last week. Apparently the delusions increased, and without going into any real detail, it was clearly the best decision from the health care professionals, at least now she will get the care and treatment that she needs, and it will also give her a break from her difficult circumstances surrounding her home and relationships.

In a strange way I almost feel pleased. I think I just feel that it was the best thing for her, and I think it has made me realise that in fact I was seeing her become very ill the week before, and in some ways this has made the way I was feeling last week more concrete, and it proves that my thoughts were correct. I thought she didn't seem well last week, and now that she is in the hospital this somehow gives some clarity to the situation that seemed to be bubbling away the week before. I don't wish to sound like I'm happy about it, because she was a well liked member of the group and I got on well with her in previous weeks, but at the same time I think I'm realising that sometimes hospital is the best place for people and now she can at least have time to get herself well again.

I had a great opportunity to speak to the manager today about healthy eating! I finally broached the subject and basically asked why there were simply no healthy food options anywhere!! Well to my surprise he said he had tried a number of times to introduce healthy foods and educate the service users, he had even got people in from the local health centre to come and give a talk on eating and health! He said it was a huge challenge, and many of the users simply were not interested.

I explained that I'm quite into healthy eating myself and that there is huge amounts of evidence to back up the claims that eating healthy can improve people's moods as well as their physical health. He was very understanding of this, and said that myself and my colleague were welcome to try and come up with any ideas that may help educate the group, but he warned me that it would be a considerable challenge! At least he has tried, but I'm now left wondering how on earth you motivate people to try new things and understand the importance of health and mood!

This could be an interesting little assignment for us! Even if it's just for a day, we could maybe at least try and educate the group. It felt good to get the topic talked about anyway, and I came away feeling a bit more positive, but at the same time a little disheartened, as I realised that it would be a huge challenge. I realised this even more as I saw the service users take their cans of pop and bars of chocolate for snacks throughout the day!!

The service user's child was in again today. I have mentioned him before, the one who consistently feeds his daughter jam sandwiches and biscuits, it was the same again today, and then there was surprise when she couldn't eat her lunch. I agreed with my student colleague that it wasn't in our place to say anything, but we didn't agree with it, I'm also a bit wary and unsure as to how safe it is to bring a child into such an environment.

I know I've mentioned it before, but I think I've started to think about things a little more now, having been here a few weeks, especially as the manager sometimes has to go to the bank, and we are left on our own. The whole group is self led, so I'm starting to think what if something happened to this guy's daughter, and she got caught up in something? She's only 18 months old, and there have been rows and fights in the past, surely this is not a good environment? But at the same time I see the joy on the service user's face when he is playing with his daughter, and today he uttered the words: *'I've had a shit life you know, but she makes it worth living, I'm really lucky aren't I?'* That said it all to me really, his daughter was the only thing keeping this guy going, and I suddenly felt guilty for having the thoughts of how he should be bringing her up as regards her health. These thoughts only fleetingly appeared, but they still made me think, I'm only thinking of the best interests of his daughter, so she can have a healthy and fulfilled life, but those words did bring me crashing into reality. I can't understand what it's like to have a child, and I also can't understand what it's like to have a mental illness, but what I could start to appreciate in front of my eyes is how a child can make people stable and provide a purpose for someone's life, and this guy readily admitted it; if it wasn't for his daughter, what would his life be like ? This is what keeps him going day after day.

On a lighter note, something else happened today that I simply couldn't really prepare myself for, our training certainly doesn't anyway; I met a lady today who apparently used to be a nurse herself until her mental health problems got in the way of her job.

Sometimes I come away from this placement simply thinking that all I've done is sit around, have a few chats to people and drink lots of cups of tea, however there are times when I start to analyse things a little more, and start to realise that may seem to be what I do on the surface, but there is a lot more to it. I've realised even writing this diary how much more I seem to be looking and thinking about things. If I am simply sitting there and having a cup of tea with someone then I would think no more of it, but I'm now beginning to realise how THAT person may see the situation, and from their point of view it may be the only contact they get all day. To sit and chat with someone might be a huge point in their day, where they can feel wanted and have someone to talk about their problems or simply what they have been doing. I think the little things make a huge difference, and I am starting to think that my time isn't wasted here; even if I only get to speak to a few people in the day, that can still be a lot of progress, and over time that can build up a rapport and make people feel more comfortable.

Just before I end the entry, I just must briefly mention that I had a good discussion with the manager about how a charity was run and set up, and how they get grants to buy various items such as furniture and equipment. I felt that it was important to break away a bit from the group today and begin to find out a bit more about how an organisation like this works. I found it very useful and valuable, and it's given me more of a rounded knowledge base. The manager has been quite supportive today and he has given me good advice. I think today has been a good day. I sometimes think too much about my purpose here, but it seems once I step back a little I begin to see how things fit together, and how people interact. I think I should just relax a little more around people and just take each situation as it comes. I think I'm finding my feet more anyway.

11/2

Today was a University day, however one of my student colleagues had arranged to go and meet a local group, it was a group for people suffering with mental distress. I hadn't heard of them before, but thought it was a good opportunity to go and visit and I could use this information to put in my database. I managed to find the place OK, and realised that I had been to the centre before, but a long time ago. Once we arrived we didn't seem to know where everyone was, in one room it was full of elderly men and women playing cards, and I was quite sure it wasn't that room!

Eventually we walked into a huge hall which had just a tiny table at the far end, and about four women sat at it knitting. This was the group!! We introduced ourselves. My student colleague already knew one of the members of the group so she was able to strike up a conversation quite easily; I recognised one of the members from the hospital. I don't think she remembered me though. I had seen her a few times, and also at the University where she had talked about her illness. I felt a bit awkward initially, it seemed to be primarily a knitting group, not my favourite subject at school! I managed to discuss with one of the main organisers of the group about what it was all about. The people there were very friendly, I was the only man there, which did feel pretty strange to me, even stranger when everyone was knitting and talking about what they had made the week before. I assumed from this that the group was all female, but apparently they did have some males who entered the group on different days, and apparently they had 'male activities' such as woodwork. I felt this was a bit sexist, not all men like woodwork and clichéd perceived 'manly tasks' but I figured I wasn't going to say anything, I'd just sit here and get a feel for the group.

Got talking to the service user that I recognised, and managed to strike up a good chat about University and how I was getting on. She didn't recognise me at all, I guess when I saw her at the hospital she was quite ill and paranoid, I didn't expect her to remember me from being at University, as this was quite a long time ago. She came in to one of the 'taster' winter schools that I attended, when I was thinking about going into mental health, so in a way she helped form my decision to start the course. I wasn't going to explain this to her, I didn't feel it appropriate, and besides I wouldn't expect anyone to remember me from so long ago! She seemed quite friendly, and interested in what I was getting up to though.

That was about it for today, got a good understanding of another group, and how it meant a lot to the people who visited. They could get on with their knitting and have a good chat and a cup of tea and catch up with friends. All in all not a bad day. My student colleague even had a go at doing some knitting for them. I had to decline about ten times, and tried to explain that if they let me loose on any of their knitting they would have to spend a whole day undoing it all! I really don't like things like that, I was awful at school and hated every minute of it, I just wouldn't feel comfortable. They found it quite amusing that I didn't want to knit, I guess being the only man there I had no one to back me up with my reasons, but it was all taken in good spirits.

5/2

<u>McMurphy</u>: **'I must be crazy to be in a loony bin like this.'**

(One Flew Over the Cuckoo's Nest, 1975)

Today we had been invited along to Voluntary to have a farewell lunch for one of the volunteers that had worked there, one of the main volunteers in charge of us (I say this in the loosest sense) and responsible for supporting us. I decided not to mention the irony of the word 'support' as I felt we certainly hadn't had any real support at all, I also found it strange that we were being invited, as we hadn't really seen much of this worker except for the odd brief chat during our weeks at Voluntary. Oh well, we even had a letter to request our presence for this lunch and if we could bring something for the lunch!

I cleverly took along some packets of crisps that I had been trying to get rid of since Christmas, as I simply don't like the flavour and want to get my house rid of unhealthy snacks. Kill two birds with one stone I thought, that and the fact that I was simply too broke to buy some cakes or other such goodies. I assumed that there would be a lot of people there and maybe some service users. When I turned up, I was very wrong indeed! It seemed that this was going to be a meeting and a lunch. They had not mentioned about a meeting in the letter. There were about six people from Voluntary, including the worker who was leaving. After we had arranged all the snacks and goodies out on the main table we all sat down and they began their meeting. After about ten minutes or so one of the volunteers said **'are you understanding all this?'** and another one said **'who are you?'** Something which I dread ever being asked, it makes you feel rather small and insignificant. I was also a bit angry that our 'support' worker hadn't actually explained or introduced us to any of the other members. It was clear to me that she was leaving and didn't really care about such trivial things. Maybe that's just my cynicism kicking in, but that's what I felt, we had to explain we were students, and after that the volunteers began explaining why they had these meetings and some of the problems that came along with it, the main one being that they couldn't get enough volunteers, or enough people to attend these meetings. As the meeting progressed I continued to feel a bit misplaced. I thought I was just here for a lunch and a goodbye. My student colleagues looked equally dismayed. One of my colleagues had to meet someone so she was getting a bit anxious with the time, and eventually the meeting did come to a close and we were able to say our goodbyes. One of my colleagues had got the support worker a leaving card and signed it from us all. I thought that was nice of her, but again I didn't feel it necessary for such an act as I didn't feel supported throughout this placement, and I didn't feel I knew the support worker enough to give her a card. I know it's a nice gesture, but I found the whole thing slightly hypocritical. I just wanted to get out of there at the end, I felt awkward, I didn't have anything to eat as most of it was just junk party food, and to top it all off we sat in on a meeting that we weren't really part of or could even understand. We might as well have sat in on a meeting spoken in Dutch for all I seemed to get out of it, most of it was a good moan about not having enough volunteers, and not being able to attract enough volunteers to work for Voluntary, somewhat ironic I thought, if they don't support us in our volunteering then how on earth are people going to stay!

Maybe it was just me, but I didn't feel like I achieved anything today, it seemed a big waste of time. I realised how big a waste of time it was when I started comparing which was the best Lethal Weapon film over and over in my head (clearly number 1, fact fans!) My attention had clearly wandered...

6/2

'I found it hard, it's hard to find, oh well whatever never mind'

(Smells Like Teen Spirit, Nirvana)

Didn't go to other placement today, I had some training to do at Voluntary! Strange hours too, 3.15pm – 6pm. I had no idea what to expect, and to top it all off, I will have to do a whole day of training the following week, oh well, without this training they won't let me work with **ANY** of their service users, so I'll have to grin and bear it. When I turned up I was one of the last people to arrive. There were quite a few people there. I had to sign in and get a name sticker to attach to myself, oh no! I hate things like this, I imagined it was going to be a whole afternoon of 'Hi, my name's Jack and I am...' and all that small talk getting to know you stuff. I've done it loads of times before, and it never gets any easier, so this didn't cheer me up.

Everyone was sat on the back row so I had no choice but to sit right at the front. I thought things couldn't get much worse, still I had a cup of green tea with me that I was allowed to make, so this cheered me up for a fraction of a second (note, intentional sarcasm). I saw my other student colleague but she was on the back row and talking to some other people. I was just sat on my own, at the front, feeling very out of place and anxious! After a while a few more people came to sit down. Rather interestingly the next person to arrive was an older chap and he chose to sit two chairs away from me. I thought this very strange, but then I thought back to my psychology interests and began comparing this behaviour to the well known patterns of behaviour from within a male urinal, the standard pattern being that the next bloke to come in will always go to the farthest urinal possible from you (See Middlemist, Knowles & Matter ,1976 for further information). Anyway, I digress, but this train of thought kept me from feeling as anxious, and I found it very interesting that this chap would sit far away from me. Luckily right before the training was to start a young female sat next to me, phew I thought, maybe I don't smell after all.

The training kicked off with a bit of small talk from the organisers, standard stuff really, what to do if there's a fire, and a bit about the organisation. We had an itinerary of what was going to happen this afternoon, it sounded OK, and look what was happening at 4pm!! A doctor was coming in for an hour, and not just any doctor, a doctor who I had been to see many times at the hospital when he gave lectures to us students, and he was brilliant! I really enjoyed his lectures so was really pleased he was coming along, he has a brilliant style and I find him very interesting to listen to, and I feel you learn a lot.

After a few brief talks from the organisers, the doctor came in and gave his talk, and as I expected, it was very informative and very interesting. After he had finished he came up to me and said he recognised me from the hospital. I said I had attended many of his lectures and thanked him for coming today. After this a small tea break, although I didn't go for a tea break, instead I started chatting to the girl next to me, she was going to do a Psychology degree and she was joining Voluntary to gain some experience, so I filled her in on what my course was like and how I got into the course, coincidentally also from an interest in Psychology. I felt pleased that I had talked to at least one other person in the group.

After the short tea break it was just a simple wrap up talk about expenses and how to claim them, standard stuff, and then that was it! No introductions, no group work, no role plays, all that was to come to my horror as I looked in my newly acquired bright blue folder which had a plan of all the rest of the training days and what they entailed!! Oh well, I have to do it, hopefully it won't be as bad as I make out in my head.

What we hadn't been told is that there were two extra evenings of training if we wanted to do befriending. I was interested in this, but I thought that this would all be encompassed in the whole day of training, but no, it's two extra evenings! And once that's done then I get a certificate to put in my portfolio! I think things are a bit of a strange way round, not being able to work with Voluntary's service users for two months, then do the training, and then be able to work with them, only by that time I'll be back in University doing lectures and in the skills labs, and won't have many weeks to actually work side by side with a volunteer. I guess Voluntary can't help when their training days are, but I wish they would have explained this at the interview. I don't think I'm going to get enough experience at this rate, I guess they figure that we can volunteer not just in term time, but at the minute I don't see how I could ever fit volunteering in alongside my training as well as doing my other placements. Sure it would be nice to do, but I simply don't have enough free time to warrant this, and I think it would cause extra anxieties and stresses. Oh well, it's difficult to say now, but it just seems a strange placement at the minute.

Get home and my student colleague texts me to say that another college wants us to do a talk to 22 of their students! Oh no!!!!!!! This has not cheered me up at all!!!!!

7/2

Due to our impending presentations, it was time to meet up at one of our colleague's houses and work out what the hell we were going to do!! The presentation at the college was on the 19th Feb., AGHHHHH! I've just looked at the date now!

Oh, hang on, I've just made a stupid error, for some reason I'm writing this entry down as the 14th February, but it's actually the 7th! I breathe a massive sigh of relief. The presentation isn't that far away, but at least its further away than I thought! Ha-ha. We have also decided on the menu to do our lunch idea, I made an executive decision and decided that we should make vegetarian chilli con carne, bosh some pans about Jamie Oliver style, and we could get people involved in chopping lots of fresh veg up if they wanted to, bung it all in a pan and heat up, serve with some wholegrain rice, that should do the trick. We had five names on the board when we checked last, so with us that makes eight people, and eight **PEOPLE** make a lunch! (And five **PEOPLE** make a conspiracy... only Nicolas Cage fans will get this reference.) Again we needed to sort a date out for this, aghhh, so many things to sort out!

12/2

Today I am going to Voluntary to meet and get briefed on a potential befriendee. All of a sudden Voluntary are very keen to get me to work with some of their service users. As my training is looming, I guess they want to strike whilst the iron is hot. I'm still unsure as to what to expect, and I feel it's still going to be a bit late in the proceedings to start all this, but hey, I figure it's got to be worth it, and I DO want to work with service users, after all that's what we're here for, right?

I decide to get myself prepped for the occasion, by blasting out some Foo Fighters on the car stereo, some loud rock to start the day. Once I get to Voluntary I have a briefing about this guy I'm potentially going to be working with; some evidence of paranoid thoughts, and hearing voices, and also a low level of Aspergers syndrome, apparently the service user's main goal is simply to make some new friends and socialise more. From scanning his case history we seem to have a few things in common, I think it might be OK, what I find strange is that our new 'support' worker is very keen to busily get me involved in things, but I fear it could all be too late. After looking through the first person's case history she says she has someone else in Voluntary for me for telephone befriending! I start to worry at this point and think how am I going to fit all this work in around my University studies?

The support worker says she has to quickly draft up a contract for both parties so that we can sign them when we go and visit him. I thought this was a bit presumptuous! What if he doesn't want to work with me? I raise the point that it's a bit forward to ask someone on the spot whether or not they want to work with someone. Isn't that putting just a bit of pressure on people to just say yes? The support worker says that she has never had a case of people saying no (well, that didn't surprise me, how many people would feel comfortable saying no, in front of the person that is supposed to be there to befriend them!), so basically she had decided we were going to work together no matter what it seemed! I suggested wouldn't it be best to ask him after I had visited, just to get a clearer idea of whether he wanted to start up the befriending. She didn't understand where I was coming from and simply stated again that there should be no problem and she had to draft up this contract before we went!

After she had prepared the contract she did ask me briefly about our progress with other aspects of our placement. I explained about the presentations we had got lined up and the cooking event. She recorded all this in her diary and then asked who was supporting us now that the other employee had left. I had to chuckle to myself, I thought she was our support worker in front of me!! I kind of stuttered and stated very sheepishly 'err no one really, we have just been self directed and getting on with our own things', she said that was not very good. What an understatement! At this point she called in one of the main guys in the office, the same guy who earlier in our placement had looked down on us as though we were mere spots of dust on the carpet, again he had this same expressionless look about him and seemed like he was being interrupted from having a very important cup of tea. The support worker asked him who was in charge of the students, he looked at me, then at the support worker, then in the most begrudging and downright miserable voice I have possibly ever heard, he simply uttered **'well.......I suppose it will have to be me.'** Charming! Well that made me feel better, thanks a lot! I quickly said that I would email him the plan of what we were doing (probably leave it a good couple of days, just so he can forget who we are again) and he sort of grunted at me, and went back in the office, which made me feel very pleased. The support worker seemed oblivious to his body language and attitude, and sort of said in a cheery smiley way 'well that's good then, you know where you are now' as though that made everything better! God, could it get much worse here!?

Well it was time to head out to the befriendee. It wasn't far and the support worker was going to drive me there, have a little chat and see how things went (although it was quite clear from her perspective that we WERE going to work together as she was clutching the forms eagerly in her hand, I wonder if she gets paid commission for every befriendee?) I was starting to feel a little nervous. I had met lots of service users before, but I think that air of nervousness will always crop up, you never quite know what to expect I guess. Walking out to the car, in the back of my mind I was thinking her car must be one of these Fiestas or Astra's parked up, all of a sudden I hear the clunk of a car opening, someone's

Audi TT was being unlocked, hang on, we were walking to this Audi TT! It was her car! A convertible shiny red Audi TT, what the hell was going on!   I didn't expect that, clearly working at Voluntary pays well!

'You're not the car you drive'

(Fight Club, 1999)

I was being briefed again in the car over the hum of the loud engine. It seemed like we could have quite a lot of things in common, as we were 'about the same age', well three years difference, but that shouldn't matter too much.

When we got to his flat, there was already his support worker there from the early intervention psychosis team. It was quite a small flat, but instantly I began to pick up on a few interests, there was a mountain bike in the lobby, and a Playstation 3 in the lounge. Good start, we might be able to have a few things in common to work with I thought. There wasn't much room in the flat, so the support worker had to sit on the floor. We had a brief chat, and then she thrust the contracts right in our faces to sign, and then said we should go for a walk to get to know each other, again an odd way round, it's almost like 'you've signed the contracts now, go and get to know him, and get on with each other.' I felt really sorry for the chap, I felt he was being put under pressure, I explained this to him as we walked round his estate and got a bit more of an idea of his interests. He seemed compliant with everything I was suggesting and didn't seem to want to know anything about me. I even asked him if he wanted me to tell him anything. I guess it was a first meeting and building rapport was going to take time. After we came back I arranged to meet him next week for a coffee, and take it from there really. I could see there were some definite social issues, but if I could get him to open up a bit when we went for coffee that should work out OK.

I had to go back to the office for a debriefing, and then I was told all about my potential telephone befriendee, just someone who wants a chat now and again apparently, it was that simple. I said I would give it a go, but again explained how my time would be limited and how I did have a holiday coming up. Once again the support worker seemed oblivious and just kept going on about how I needed to make a commitment, which is fine in principal but I cannot let my University work suffer as a result, but I agreed, cos I figure it can't hurt to try these things and I still have about three weeks to work at

Voluntary. I couldn't start or speak to this new person until I had done my training, so we just left it for now, and the support worker was going to arrange it all for after my training had been completed. All in all quite an interesting day, at least I did something constructive and made contact with an actual service user, although I'm starting to feel guilty about how much time I can offer him, and I don't think that the people at Voluntary understand our University time commitments, I just feel it's going to be a case of meeting up with him for a few coffees and then it will be time to move on to another placement, and I don't want to feel guilty about this. University has to be the priority, if I fall behind there then I'm not working with anyone full stop!

13/2

"I gotta say it was a good day, didn't even have to use my A.K'
Ice Cube

Back to the other placement today. I really don't feel like it, I can't put my finger on why, maybe it's the cold weather, I just want to stay in bed and let the world pass me by today, but I don't, I get up and make my way there. When I get there, there are some huge construction vehicles and a JCB knocking down the old pub next door. As a result of this, there is no parking anywhere! I drive past where I normally park, I can see another building in the distance next to the placement, I hastily drive down a very narrow lane. I think this lane is actually for pedestrians, but in my haste I just carry on down it, and park up next to another car. God knows how I am going to get back out of here, but at least my car was parked!

When in the building, there were the same familiar faces, I said hello, and got a cup of tea. My other student colleague was already there, and I sat and chatted to her for a bit. There didn't seem as many people here today. We were talking about how it would be good to do something to get out of the building. I commented that I thought every Wednesday was a walking day, and a lot of the members went in their car and went for a walk round the area. It was time to take action, we wanted to be involved! So I quickly spoke to the manager and asked if we could go along. No problem. This was a turn up for the books, we were actually going to get properly involved in something and not feel constrained to just one building!

We followed some of the other people who were going in their car. When we got to the area there was a huge gathering of people! I had assumed it was only going to be the few people from the placement going, but apparently this was a proper organised event! And it happened most weeks, sometimes more than once a week, well that was a surprise, we even had to register. Initially I felt a bit out of place; we were the youngest people there by a long way, but I soon got into the swing of things the walk was a scarily looking '3 hearts' which ranks it as a middle ranking walk, to last an hour. I envisaged huge sprawling masses of hills and climbing, but then I suddenly realised I was in reality, and that these walks weren't supposed to be back breaking and gruelling, it was just a nice walk around the area at a nice gentle pace.

The walk only lasted an hour, but it was literally and figuratively a breath of fresh air. I really enjoyed it, and got to chat to the organisers (or walk leaders as their official title claimed, due to the imprinting of this on the back of their fluorescent jackets) and the walk even went through a market and car boot sale, which was just designed to tempt me to buy more stuff to sell on eBay, but I managed to resist, and kept up with the group.

The walks happen most weeks so I and my student colleague agreed that we should do this more often as it made a nice change from the norm. When I got back, I met up with a few other people I knew who were playing pool. I asked if I could have a game afterwards, to which the one guy agreed, this was more like it! I was having a good day so far, and now I was going to play pool finally. The guy I was playing managed to successfully lose the game twice in one go, as he potted the black once, then we played on, and then he did it again! We had a good chuckle about this, and everyone's spirits seemed high. I felt more relaxed this time, maybe because I was chatting to people I had built up a bit of rapport with, but I didn't feel uncomfortable, and we all had a good chat and a bit of fun.

After the pool (we played two games, and drew) it was time to just have another cup of tea and a chat. I was speaking to a chap who used to travel all around the world doing web programming for international clients, it sounded really interesting, he then began to tell me all about his experiences about the hospital and how he escaped the one day and got as far as seven miles! He was able to have a joke about his experiences but he did have a more serious tone and said how he would never want to go back to the hospital and he said how ill he was, he was complaining of having a dry mouth, so my colleague suggested a glass of water, but he went for another can of coke zero. I tried to subtly explain to him how caffeine works on the human body and can in effect dehydrate him, he didn't quite seem to take this on board but said he drank a lot of water at home, I didn't want to push him into not having a particular drink, but merely subtly suggest why maybe coke isn't necessarily the best drink to keep having if you are feeling thirsty. I thought it's his decision at the end of the day but it can't hurt to shoehorn in a bit of health promotion! I was really enjoying myself today, everything seemed to be going really well, and the people I talked to seemed to be quite jokey and able to have a laugh. I almost regretted leaving today, but I really had to press on with other things. I felt much more comfortable with my surroundings and felt I had made a difference today.

13/2 (7:30pm)

After taking an obscene amount of eBay packages to the post office, it was time to get ready to go out again. I was meeting another student colleague in town and we were going to a group which meets up weekly, and whose members consist of people with Aspergers syndrome. Tonight they were meeting in the pub. I thought this would be an excellent opportunity to get to meet some new people, and as my befriendee had low levels of Aspergers I thought this might eventually be a good group for him to get involved in, so I needed to suss it all out first, and it was meeting in a pub, so I figured that was a good venue to start with.

When we turned up at the pub, there was only one person there. I was unsure as to how many people would be attending, but as the minutes passed more and more people started coming in. We made our introductions and began to talk to some of the people there. They seemed interested that we were student nurses. I initially felt like a bit of an outsider, crashing the party so to speak but eventually everyone made us very welcome, and the one chap had a Heroes t shirt on, so my colleague was instantly able to spark up a bit of a conversation about this and other related TV shows. Within about half an hour there were a good fifteen people in the pub, and the main organiser who ran it was sat next to me, so she was able to fill me in on a few details.

It was an interesting night, it felt good to get out and speak to new people, I think it gains my confidence more and also broadens my scope of knowledge. The group are trying to organise a bowling night the start of next month, and they seemed quite keen for us to attend, so I think I will try and make that, plus it's an ideal location as I can walk up there!

15/2

A whole day training at Voluntary! I wasn't looking forward to this today. When I got to the building I had a text from my other student colleague who was supposed to be coming along, she said she was ill and wasn't turning up! I felt awful! I was looking forward to her coming along for a bit of moral support, but now I realised I was going to be left on my own. I didn't feel overly comfortable with many of the people there as I didn't know them, oh well I was going to have to combat these anxieties on my own, and just get through the day! I was already quite knackered by the time I arrived as I had decided to bike down to Voluntary, in an effort to keep fit and keep the costs down on my petrol.

The start of the day seemed OK, it consisted of a talk by someone from the Samaritans. There was a lot of group work almost right from the start, the first one being just to chat to the person next to you, and once the guy giving the talk coughed I had to look disinterested in what the other person was saying, look distracted, and break eye contact, just to prove how important body language is in listening and communication skills.

Most of this I already kind of knew. I had previously done a diploma in body language and a lot of the skills I needed for that course were employed in most of today's role plays.

During the afternoon we had another speaker. We had met this speaker before, and she was a woman who must be in her eighties I guessed. I felt quite concerned at one point that I might have to try and remember my resuscitation techniques as she seemed quite shaky as she drank her cup of tea. I thought she was going to 'go' right there and then, her voice was actually trembling! The room was silent, I could feel a tense nervousness in the air from everyone else sat there, you could hear the faint chinking of the cup hitting the saucer. I felt everyone else in the room sort of lean forward in anticipation, the chinking of the cup got more frequent... until eventually she managed to put it down on a nearby table. Everyone sat back in their seats, I thought please don't faint now, I don't know enough to help if something goes wrong! But luckily she was strong throughout and she knew her stuff to be fair, and got us involved in all sorts of group work and activities, some of it more embarrassing than others!

At one point I had to pretend I was a new volunteer to the group and introduce myself to a group of the rest of the volunteers who were pretending to be service users. It felt quite awkward and stilted at times, but I guess there was an underlying theme and some learning going on! I just don't always like the feel of role play, it makes me feel a bit self conscious at times and unnatural. I understand it is trying to shape your learning but it doesn't always seem to come off like that for me!

By the end of the day I was quite drained. We got through an awful lot of training, and a lot of role plays. I didn't detest the day as I thought I would, but in some sense came away thinking about some of the skills that we had discussed and felt it gave me a better understanding. It's strange, sometimes I make things out to be a lot worse in my head, and they usually turn out not so bad in reality. I wouldn't say it was a lot of fun, but It did make me think, and some of the skills talked about were extremely valid and would be of use throughout my future placements and career.

18/2

<u>Joel Goodson</u>: **You know, Bill, there's one thing I learned in all my years. Sometimes you just gotta say, "What the fuck, make your move."**

(Risky Business, 1983)

Before going to the Voluntary training, myself and my other student colleagues had a meeting booked with one of the lecturers. We were going to discuss how unhappy we were working with Voluntary, and more importantly how much stress we felt we were being put under by them. The meeting went well, and I think we got our point across well. It felt good to discuss it with someone from the University, and the lecturer understood some of the points we were making. A lot of the time we felt we were being treated more as students rather than volunteers, and thought that many of the activities we were being asked to get involved with would not be activities that Voluntary would get their normal volunteers to engage in. It's difficult to separate the student stigma from being a volunteer, and we feel maybe this is where it was going wrong. We explained how hard it was to approach the staff at Voluntary, and felt that they couldn't really listen to us or understand our other prior commitments such as our University work.

The lecturer suggested writing everything down in an email and the lecturer would then write to Voluntary subtly explaining our concerns, and hopefully get a better understanding that way and maybe improve things, the main reason being that we felt under obligation and pressure to work within our annual leave. Voluntary would simply say that it's only an hour a week, and a chat and a coffee. Whilst this in principal is fine, it's not just that, it's the travel into town, and the travel back, and I think it's the principle of the fact that our annual leave is supposed to be a break away from everything!

I don't feel comfortable in working through my annual leave and nor do any of the other students, so between us we wrote quite possibly the biggest email in the universe and got all our thoughts down! This made us feel a lot better, and maybe some good will come of it, or maybe it will all end in tears and bloodshed! Well, something had to be done, maybe we left it too late, but at least we have gone and done something and that helped clear my and my colleagues' minds.

It was good to get our thoughts down, and we felt pleased we had done this email, as we thought it needed to be written down and sent.

The day however wasn't over, it was time for more training! This time at 5.30pm till 8pm, and it was on befriending. Since I had already arranged to have a meeting with my befriendee the following day I needed to go to this, unfortunately most of it was exactly what I had been told the previous week, so I found the whole thing a little boring. We got to watch a video, but it turned out it was the video we were using in our presentation for the college, so we had already seen it! So that wasn't exactly a good start, although it wasn't a particularly long video, and afterwards there were a few questions on the video about what we thought about it. I didn't really say anything, I was a bit tired from the day's activities. I found some of the things the staff at Voluntary were saying were contradicting themselves, particularly as I had spent all afternoon writing that email slagging off a lot of their 'support' networks. I didn't feel very supported at all, and a lot of the training tonight seemed to centre around how supported volunteers would feel, how ironic!

To top it all off, after the training, we couldn't get out of the car park, trapped here forever! Both gates were closed, so we had to go back in, grab the final two staff and plead with them to let us out as we didn't want to spend all night in my car in the freezing cold. Luckily they let us out (although if they had read my email from before to the lecturer they may have thrown away the keys forever and kept us trapped in the car park).

Tonight just felt like a bit of a rambling on about nothing. When we went back into Voluntary to get someone to let us out, I overheard one of the staff say 'was it all right tonight?' I just made most of it up on the spot'. Well that just made things quite clear to me there and then! I felt I couldn't trust these people and there was an air of insincerity about them, I just wanted to leave as quickly as I could, I had had enough of them for today, I felt the whole thing a bit of a waste of time and semi patronising, and didn't feel I had learnt anything today that's for sure, the lecture just seemed to paint a picture of a perfect world where everyone was supported and looked after, and I was already sensing that this might not be the case at all!

19/2

<u>Jerry Maguire</u>: **Jump in my nightmare, the water's warm!**

(Jerry Maguire, 1996)

Oh god! Have to do a presentation this morning, to a group of kids, I'm not looking forward to it at all. I thought I had already done the presentation earlier this morning, but realised that unfortunately it was all just a dream. I couldn't sleep well throughout the night either, I felt a bit better after a pint of freshly juiced carrots and apples, and thought that I should be OK, but then I was thinking I might feel a bit more nervous once I actually got there, oh well, at least we were going to do it as a team, I think I would go to pieces if it was just me on my own!

I met up with my student colleague and off we went to the college. When we got to the reception, there was no sign of the teacher we were supposed to see! One of the women on reception said she thought the teacher worked over at the other part of the college. A sense of unease dawned on us; the teacher had never stated which campus she wanted us to do the presentation in!! It was 8.25am, we were supposed to be meeting the teacher at 8.15am, and we were already 10 minutes late and at the wrong campus! I started to feel sick, part of me foolishly thought 'oh well, they will have to cancel it now' but this thought only lasted a few seconds, because by then we were racing out of the building, jumping in my car and about to put pedal to metal and speeding down to the other campus! This was quite difficult in places, as today has been one of the coldest days ever and there seems to be an awful lot of eerie mist everywhere, particularly around the roundabouts, so I had to be quite careful.

Eventually turned up at the correct reception! And just as we got there the teacher turned up herself! That was good timing; we weren't late after all. We thought we could get away with not telling her about our foolish error of going to the wrong campus (but to be fair she hadn't indicated which one to go to either, she had just assumed like us) but before we could hide this fact, the receptionist blurted it out, and we all laughed. She did apologise, but it was all taken quite light heartedly. The teacher was very nice and showed us to the classroom. Everything was set up, projector and laptop, it was going to be OK I thought, there were no students present at the minute, we just had a bit of time to set up our gear, and then we were told to come back about half an hour later and get ready to do our presentation!

We went to the cafeteria for a quick cup of tea. I was starting to panic now, it all felt so real. I actually liken this feeling to queuing up to go on a rollercoaster, I'm usually fine for most of it, but when I'm actually about to sit in the coaster and get strapped in that's when I start feeling my stomach go and feel the nerves fly (although I do love roller coasters, I don't love presentations!). I was trying to keep my nerves under wraps. My other colleagues didn't seem as nervous as me, unless they were all hiding them too!

Not long to go now, it was time to finish up our cup of tea and walk back along the corridor and up the stairs.

We waited outside patiently. The teacher had seen us, the classroom was full of students, all women it seemed, I suddenly realised that it was all going to happen now within moments! I just wanted to jump out of the window! (Or something else less damaging maybe!) I was two people away from sitting on Oblivion (Alton Towers, Staffordshire, the world's first vertical drop roller coaster fact fans!) I thought this is it in a minute, as soon as I go through those classroom doors that's it, I'm sitting on Oblivion, strapped in, and can't get off, and this was going to be a ride of total fear or enjoyment, or a mix of both.

The classroom door opened, the teacher led us through, and we walked right to the front of the classroom, where there were about 25 students eyes all staring at us, and they were all women, not a male in sight! (Click click click goes the ride, starting its ascent up the track.)

My heart started to pound a bit but I tried to keep it in check. The teacher did a little introduction for us. (Oblivion is slowly making its way round the top of the track, curving around towards the eventual pivot over the impending drop.)

And then it was over to us. I was going first, I was introducing us all, and I was speaking first, this was it! (Oblivion pivots and holds over the drop for three seconds, a creepy voice utters **'DON'T LOOK DOWNNNN'**, and then the catches release and woooooshh, straight down into the black pit, stomach is lost)

I just went for it. I had to fight these nerves, I think I was doing all right, I noticed some of the girls smiling, this put me off, I thought I was sounding really nervous. I heard my colleague whispering behind me, this made me even more paranoid, was I doing something wrong? Was I not saying the right things? I soldiered on, I missed a few things off my PowerPoint, but I couldn't go back now, I just had to do the best I could. I felt I stumbled through some of it, but I couldn't help it, I had forgotten how nerve racking presentations could be. I tried to find my calm, and I think I managed to level myself out a bit, I don't think it helped that they were all young female students, and a few were smiling and laughing to themselves. I take this to be a sign of disinterest and that just puts me off even more. I wish I could have said more now, but I finally came to an end and passed on to my other colleague, it was done now. (Oblivion comes up through the black hole, turns and the air brakes kick in, a sense of relief comes over me). I felt angry with myself, I think I could have done better, It could have been a lot smoother, but sometimes these nerves just come from nowhere, I hope I didn't appear to nervous on the outside, I just felt like leaving the room now and going home!

After everyone had said their bit it was time for a few questions from the teacher, and some of the students started to have their own questions which I think we all managed to answer quite well, there was also some interest in what it was like to be a student nurse as some of the class were interested in going into nursing, so again we were able to explain this quite successfully, after that it was time to take a few pictures to prove we actually did it, although I can't quite believe that I made it! I found the questions and answering part of the presentation much more relaxing and felt more comfortable, I think it's just the very nature of a presentation and being up there for everyone to listen to.

And then it was time for us to go. One of the students thanked us, I'm not sure how many of the others appreciated it, but it was all done now, we wouldn't see them again, but I just hope we did make some impact on some of them, otherwise it would be a huge waste of time. The teacher seemed very pleased though and even invited us back another time if we wanted to (at this point I very much didn't want to come back!) Oh well, at least we achieved something, it was hard work, but I feel I got through it OK.

I found out afterwards that when I was doing my introduction, the talking from my student colleague was actually to the other colleague saying how she didn't think she could go through with doing her bit of the presentation, it wasn't about me at all. It made me more comfortable knowing that afterwards, and to be fair the colleague did apologise to me as I had said I got a bit paranoid and nervous because I could hear them chatting! But it was just nerves, so I wasn't the only one. At the end of the day, we are always going to be a bit nervous, but I guess the more times you do things like this the better, and to think I once thought of being a teacher! I'm not sure I could go through with that sort of pressure every single day!

After the presentation we all went our separate ways. I took the boards back to Voluntary that we had used for our presentation with one of my student colleagues, and the support worker there asked us how our presentation went. They seemed really pleased, and they also asked if we wore our Voluntary sweatshirts that we had been given!!

Small dramatic silence........

'Err no' we kind of stumbled, we said we didn't feel they were appropriate for this particular target market, or words to that effect, something that sounded professional rather than what we were actually thinking which was 'we took one look at them, they looked poor and we would feel like melons in them speaking to a load of students'. They seemed to take our professional answer well, and we did state that we would wear them for a car boot sale! So that was our saving grace really.

All in all I don't know how to rate today, I feel so glad it's over, I'm not sure whether to feel good or not, I feel a bit miserable now, and a bit angry at myself, because I feel it could have gone better, but I guess practice makes perfect. I was only annoyed at myself really, I thought the other colleagues did really well, and one of them said she wasn't nervous at all! What was her secret!! I got a nice text thanking me for putting the video onto DVD and for doing the PowerPoint for the presentation, so that cheered me up, I just hope I didn't let the team down with my nerves. Oh well; it's all good experience, and all good evidence for our portfolio!

I'm going to meet my befriendee in an hour. I feel guilty for saying it, but I'm not sure I want to go, it's more to do with the fact that I'm not sure I'm going to have enough time in weeks to see this partnership through, maybe I should see how today goes, but I'm feeling like everything is caving in on me and we have so much to do at Voluntary that things are going to get missed and I'm not going to be able to give him the full support that he needs. Maybe I should call this partnership off soon, but I will go today just to see how he is, but I cannot work in my annual leave, I simply will want a complete break for two weeks! I will see how it goes, but there is so much to be doing at the minute I just can't see how to get on top of it all.

2pm...Same day...

I arranged to meet my befriendee in the square. I turn up in the square a few minutes early, and I can't see him, I wonder around for a bit, and then I realise he is actually sitting down on one of the benches talking to someone else. I go over to him and get introduced to the chap he is sitting next to. I have no idea who this person is, but I assume it must be a friend or maybe someone he works with. The first thing I ask him is where he fancies going for a coffee, he suggests Starbucks, which is right by the square. I was fancying somewhere a bit quieter as it seemed crammed full of students, but I didn't want to upset him, I figure it should be his choice.

I made sure I ordered the 'small' cup of tea, which still seemed to resemble an absolutely HUGE mug. What has happened to the sizes of coffee mugs? TALL is the smallest, GRANDE is the medium, and VENTI is the largest! Venti means bucket! Since when did we need to consume a pint of coffee as a mid morning or afternoon drink? I smile at the frankly ludicrous size of my mug of tea.

I went to go and find my befriendee, who had already gone off and found a seat somewhere. I found him around the corner, in probably the smallest and most uncomfortable seating arrangement I had ever seen, it was right by the entrance door, and I had to kind of squeeze into a really tight space and couldn't seem to move the table at all. It was lucky I hadn't put on any weight, as it felt ridiculously cramped and awkward. I didn't feel comfortable at all, and there wasn't much space between us, so I think this was going to hamper my communication with the guy.

He started off talking about quite a few things. As I was unhooking my IPod he began to comment on how much he wanted one, and this kind of allowed us to go off into a nice casual conversation about music and technology. I thought things were going well, he also began to explain about his voices and how they were much better managed now, and that they only bothered him at some points. I was quite pleased, he was opening up a lot more, but then he kept saying how he hadn't got very long and how he had to walk home and meet his mother. Fair enough I thought, it was only going to be a quick meeting then. About halfway through the conversation everything seemed to be going OK, but then all of a sudden I encountered some abruptness.

All of a sudden I realised he was giving one word answers and he looked distracted, what was going on I thought? We had been getting on so well, but things had definitely taken a turn for the worse. As soon as I had finished my tea he stood up almost immediately and said he had to be on his way. We agreed another time to meet up next week, and that was it, he was off!

I was left wondering if that was a good meeting or not, I couldn't quite decide! Oh well, at least I had met him, and tried my best, that's all I can do really.

20/2

I had arranged to go to a third sector voluntary placement talk at the University, hoping this would be useful for our work on the database that we had to compile. It was going to be a full day, 9.30am till 4pm, but I was hoping it would be good to go to and a bit of a change, and also there would be a free lunch!!

I picked up my student colleague and I drove in, we got there in plenty of time, there was a small exhibition at the front of the building, and some of the voluntary sector were there setting up their stands, and who else was there! Two people from VOLUNTARY! So that's why they needed the boards back! Well they had never told us they were going to be at our University, when we went to say hello to them they looked incredibly sour faced and not exactly pleased to see us (the feeling's mutual I'm sure). We had a quick chat, but one of those chats where both parties weren't really interested in what each other had to say, but merely a form of small talk just designed for pleasantries, and then we were on our way. Well after that we had to go and register and oh look, get a name badge which had a designated table underneath it!! **WHAT WAS THIS ALL ABOUT!** And that wasn't the best bit, we then walked into the main area where everyone was having a cup of coffee, and most people in there were all dressed up in suits and looking highly professional. My heart sank, I didn't realise the event was so formal, and I also didn't realise that we were all going to be split up and put on different tables, oh no! This was awful, I already felt self conscious, but this made it even worse, one glance at the agenda and it clearly stated about 'group work and presentations'. Oh dear. I was going to have to work with a load of people I didn't know and pretend to know things about a subject I was just trying to learn about myself, hmmmm, this was not good! My colleague also wasn't too impressed, she was also on a different table from me, but she decided to change her table to mine, so that was one good thing, I wasn't looking forward to this! There were a few other students in the room from our group, so we talked a little bit to them before the main presentations started. I still felt a bit out of place, I had come in my normal student clothing and everyone else was all smart and in business suits (well the majority were) there was plenty of free tea and coffee, but no herbal tea! Typical, this was no good at all! I felt like leaving there and then!

We were all asked to go into the main lecture room and the day was about to begin. We found our table which was towards the front, and there were another six people on it, luckily there was one other lady who we had recognised from our meeting with the Aspergers group. Well that was a good start at least, at least there was someone we could speak to, the rest of the people on our table were mainly middle aged and in business suits and I'm not exactly sure that they even looked at us mere students, they seemed to be very snobbish and clearly not interested in us, to which the feeling appeared mutual, god I felt horrible!

The talks began, with many different speakers. Each talk was about ten minutes long, some of it was OK, but a lot of it sailed straight over my head and made me feel incredibly stupid, I guess the main points to the talks in a lot of cases were that they were trying to regulate the voluntary sector by introducing all sorts of new frameworks that voluntary bodies would have to fill in, in order to assess what areas they were doing well in, and other areas they were not, thus highlighting areas for improvement.

The talks were incredibly corporate I thought, and I didn't quite feel like I fitted in, eventually it got up to lunchtime and I decided I couldn't take it any more, I had to leave, my colleague was also leaving anyway and I agreed to give her a lift on my way back, we did explain to some of the people there that we were leaving, and they seemed fine about it, I'm sure that the people left on our table wouldn't even notice we were gone!

Just before we left we had to do some very minor group work, and the ladies just took it upon themselves to write everything themselves and discuss it amongst themselves, and when we tried to offer our opinions they didn't seem to like it at all, and almost blanked us. I just couldn't carry on like that all afternoon; I must have been serious about going as I missed out on the free lunch! But even that would have been a hassle I thought, there was a HUGE queue for the food, and knowing my luck I bet I would end up sitting with a load of suits feeling very out of place whilst they talked about corporate strategies and commissioning sectors, maybe I should have given it a chance, maybe I would have made some small talk and things would have been OK, but I had made up my mind, I didn't feel like staying and I had lots of work to get on with at home. I had made an effort to come, and I had picked up some useful leaflets but I thought this was all I could stand, so made a quick exit!

My colleague suggested a few things about my meeting with my befriendee and stated that maybe the conversation took a dip the other day because he was starting to hear his voices again. I had not thought of this, and this seemed to be a very valid point, maybe I shouldn't feel so bad about the meeting now, I had to remember that he was ill and he did hear voices still, so I couldn't rule this out, this made me feel better about the situation at least.

21/2

Telephone Befriending Training

More training!! Aghhhh, how can I cope, and another inconvenient time of 5.30pm till 8.30pm! Oh well, it was the last of the training at Voluntary at least, turned up DEAD on 5.30pm, which for some reason I felt mildly impressed with, and chuckled to myself about it, but the laughs were soon to be over as I found that everyone had migrated to the back row, and yet again I had to sit right on the front row right next to the projector screen. All was not lost because they had got a mini buffet full of sandwiches and crisps, and I was absolutely famished, my stomach was actually creaking and groaning so I was quite pleased the buffet was here!

The lady running the training introduced herself, she didn't work for Voluntary, but she did work for Age Concern, and said she had run these training sessions on numerous occasions. Tonight's training was exclusively on telephone befriending, I still wasn't sure I was actually going to work with a telephone befriendee but figured it couldn't hurt to learn about it, and might come in useful for future placements. I still felt a bit uncomfortable about sitting RIGHT at the end and RIGHT at the front, which was RIGHT next to the speaker, but I didn't have much choice, the speaker introduced herself and then suddenly started talking about the lottery and what would we do if we won 95 million pounds, she turned to me 'WHAT would YOU do with it?' I stumbled out a rather pathetic answer of 'I'd err buy ten mansions', and then she moved on to the next person in the group, and carried on till everyone had answered, it's funny what you think of when on the spot, I think what I'd really do with 95 million is initially fund a high octane action Bruckheimeresque Hollywood movie with my friends, take it to Cannes and sit on my own private yacht trying to promote it, but hey, the point of the exercise was just a little ice breaker, and it did its job.

The next item on the agenda was to make us more aware of our listening skills. We had to pair up with someone and one was to be the communicator the other the listener. I chose to be the communicator and my job was to explain to the person sitting next to me how to draw a map. They had a blank map in front of them, and I had the completed map in front of me, I basically had to describe to them what was on my map, so that they could recreate the map. I was allowed to describe the map in as many words as I wanted, and the listener could ask questions, but I could only answer these questions with a yes or a no. The exercise was OK, initially it didn't really feel that difficult, I was just describing a map, but a few points were quite tricky I guess, I ended up describing the map pretty well as it was almost faithfully recreated, a few things slightly different, but all in all a good attempt!

It did highlight some importance's of communication and also of listening, after this exercise, time to break for a cuppa!

After the break, it was mainly more talking about importance of listening and how to handle difficult calls, where people might be saying they want to commit suicide, the speaker kept me listening, as she had learnt my name AND I was on the front row, so she kept referring to me the odd times or asking me the odd question. I didn't mind this, but I did feel like I should have not been so cocky about being bang on time to the training, as if I had got here early I could have hidden in the back row!

She was a nice speaker though, and she did make some good points. The training ended about half an hour early, and before we left we were given another certificate! This was good, more evidence for the portfolio! Fantastic!

Amazingly I hadn't learned from the previous evening's training and yet again the gates were locked, so I had fun and games getting the keys this time and opening the large metal gate. At least it wasn't as cold this time. I had enjoyed the training but was glad it was all over, it was quite an intense programme of events really, but I felt more knowledgeable and it will come in handy I thought! Now I was worried that Voluntary would be ringing me up straight away trying to push a telephone befriendee on me. I'm not trying to sound like I don't want to do it, but the workload this year is quite heavy, and I don't want to put myself in a position where I'm letting my uni work suffer because I am taking on too many jobs.

I've decided I won't do the telephone befriending at this stage, but at least I've got the certificate so I know I can engage in it whenever

I feel it more suitable and when there is less pressure on me as a student (if this actually happens or not we shall have to see!)

25/2

<u>Sofía</u>: **'Every passing minute is another chance to turn it all around.'**

(Vanilla Sky, 2001)

Realised today that we hadn't got the menus from the workshop for our cooking event, so I went with my student colleague to go and pick them up. I was quite surprised when we got there, they looked really professional! I had created the menu all myself and I was pleased with how they looked, the staff at Abbey Works even commented on how they thought it was a good idea to educate and inform people about what was in their meal, rather than just put a recipe down on a bit of paper, I was well chuffed! They had also printed out my poster designs for the car boot sale, which again looked pretty impressive, they were pretty simple ideas, but I thought they looked quite eye catching. I was quite chuffed today! I could actually see some of my work in print, and they looked good, I really hope people are going to come to this cooking event now; it would be a shame if no one turned up!

The posters for the venue were very roughly knocked up, but I figured it's best to go for minimal wording and a strong use of the logo in order to stand out, quite pleased with the results, and they were blown up to A3 and laminated so they should do the trick!

Thought it was important to put the charity number on both designs just to assure people that it was a real organisation, we are planning to also have leaflets and key rings to make it look more legitimate also

26/2

The Big Cook Off!

<u>Marty McFly</u>: **'If you put your mind to it, you can accomplish anything.'**

(Back to the future, 1985)

Today was the cook off, I was wondering if anyone would actually turn up, I didn't feel like they were going to, so as I packed up all the food I was wondering how much of it would actually be used, it would be a terrible waste if no one came. I still felt that we should have met the people who wanted to go at Voluntary and walk up with them, a lot of people haven't got the confidence to go somewhere new, and if they were unfamiliar with where the hall was, then they simply wouldn't turn up.

I went and picked up my other student colleagues, they also had the same reservations, we had gone to a lot of effort with this. I didn't want things to collapse now, but it was out of our hands, we would just have to wait and see.

First problem, nowhere to park! The hall does have a car park, but it's full today, and its almost 12.30. Dammit, what are we going to do?! We quickly find a car park not too far away, but it's only a two hour stay car park! Oh dear, we are just going to have to take it in turns to come back every two hours and feed the machine with more money! We quickly parked up and I carried everything up the hill. When we got to the hall there were people waiting outside for us! That's a turn up for the books I thought, and there was also a new volunteer from Voluntary there, who I had met on the training, she was there to help us out, brilliant I thought! The more the merrier.

We quickly opened up and assessed the situation, turns out that one of the guys waiting outside was a reporter from the chronicle newspaper, he was very tight on time, and asked if he could take a quick picture of the three of us, amongst all the ingredients, we did a quick pose, and then he was off.

We had to set up the tables and chairs and look for cooking implements, for some reason I felt a little on edge as I was aware we had to get the ball rolling and wanted to get some structure sorted, I went round all the cupboards and doors and immediately panicked as I couldn't see any pots or pans, just lots of plates and dishes, where were all the pots?! There were pots when I came to visit, I thought if need be I would have to rush to my parents' house and borrow all their pots and pans, someone suggested cooking out of a tea pot! This would have worked as the teapot was quite tall, but in the end we did find some large deep pots, so we were away, I had a very quick introduction to the service users, there were three in total, and they were asking me what they could do, I felt like a proper chef! I told them I needed carrots chopping and onions, and some garlic too, this was great, everyone wanted to get involved!

We decided to get the kettle on and asked people if they wanted to try some herbal teas, a few did, but some others wanted tea and coffee. **TEA AND COFFEE!** Ahhh, big problem, in my haste of wanting to keep the day completely healthy I had neglected to actually consider getting any proper tea and coffee, I had also not purchased any milk or sugar, my student colleague came to the rescue! She went and got some whilst I carried on organising everyone.

Got my other student colleague and the volunteer to help with the banana cake, this recipe was dead simple, so I was just instructing them what I needed them to do, things were coming along nicely, one of the service users was asking me all about the chilli we were going to make and I was explaining to her how simple and easy it was to make. She seemed very interested, and I said it would keep for days and could be frozen, I actually felt like a part of something good today, I think the message was definitely getting across about healthy eating and cooking on a budget, we were on a roll.

Next problem, trying to light the enormous cooker, it seemed to have a huge ignition switch in order to light the oven. I kept clicking the button in but nothing was happening, oh god, don't tell me we can't get the oven on! After a few attempts the button suddenly sprung out, went absolutely FLYING and fell on the floor. Err, try not to panic I thought, aha! Shit, I quickly grabbed the switch and tried to figure out exactly how it went back in, the spring

Jack Bennington

was missing, so I had to sort of push it in at a very strange angle, and it looked completely cocked up, but it would have to do.

There were some strategically placed cooks long matches by the side of the cooker (hmmm, maybe the ignition switch is properly broken anyway, well it certainly is now!), I managed to get the ignition switch back into the cooker and just lit the cooker with the matches, aha, success, it was roaring away, ready to take on the banana cakes!

Whilst I was breaking the cooker, other people were setting up the chairs and tables; we even put the menus on the table to look professional.

Things were working well, people kept asking me what I wanted them to do next, I didn't feel anxious now, I felt like everything was running smoothly, and I quite enjoyed telling people what I wanted them to do. I think even my student colleague enjoyed being told how to make a banana cake.

One of the service users even had a suggestion to put grated carrots in with the banana cake, I said no problem, I hadn't done that myself, but I could see he was enjoying the freedom to alter the cake to his liking, he said he wasn't going to have any of the chilli, but he was very interested in trying the banana cake, and I said that he could make his own cake with his own design, this seemed to spur him on and encouraged him to get more involved with the process. I was glad he suggested this, I didn't want it to just be me ordering people around, I wanted the service users to think about what they were doing and enjoy the process, and hopefully take something away with them (literally and figuratively) from the day and maybe utilise some of the skills when they are back in their home environment.

I kept running about and checking up on things, two cakes were now in the oven, and the chilli was on the go, the onions were in the pots, and the garlic was about to go in. I think it was running smoothly, I couldn't sit down or stop, I felt I had to keep checking things, but I was enjoying it. I was getting a real buzz out of the activity in the kitchen, and was glad everyone was getting involved. I had to chuckle to myself as I thought of Gordon Ramsay shouting at everyone in his kitchen and telling them to move their arses, but I

132

did refrain from saying this, even in a joking manner, it would have been highly inappropriate!

We were looking round for another pot, we had got two on the go already on the cooker, but needed a larger one, all of a sudden we found one right at the back of the cupboard, it was the size of a spaceship in comparison, and we could have used that one all along! I think in all our haste we hadn't really looked properly in the back of the cupboards, this would be ideal.

A worker from Voluntary briefly turned up, I told her straight that I didn't want to do the telephone befriending and she was fine with that, she seemed pleased in what we were accomplishing but she said she couldn't stay. I thought that it was a shame but at least she could see that we were working hard.

Everything was done pretty much, but look at the time! I had to leg it down to the car and back, as I had ten minutes to go on my ticket, amazingly I ran most of the way there and back, when I got back the chilli was done, and we were about to serve up, decided we would have one big table so we could all sit around it and chat, put the chilli in bowls on the table so people could help themselves.

I felt really good about things, everyone had contributed fantastically and now we were all going to sit down and enjoy the meal. Had a really good conversation with some of the service users, chatted about how they felt they were stigmatised at times and how some people thought that just because they had a mental illness, it meant that they couldn't discuss current events or be knowledgeable about certain things, this was a good point, and one that I could learn from and take forward in my practice. I think there will always be some form of stigma around, but if we can work towards lessening it in any way we can then that can only be a good thing. It was very interesting to hear it from a service user's point of view.

Everyone said how nice the chilli was; one of the service users had four platefuls! We must be doing something right! And another of the service users said she wanted the recipe for the banana cake off me before she went! Wow, I was made up, that was really nice, I thought if she can make that on her own at home that would be a great achievement, and I have helped educate someone.

Just as we were about to finish the manager came in from Voluntary. I get a sneaky suspicion that they all want to check up on us just to see how we are doing, which is fair enough, but it would have been nicer for some of the staff to come and join us and eat, but never mind, at least he could see our efforts. He said he wanted to treat this cooking idea as a pilot scheme and maybe broaden it out to Telford and make it more regular. I thought that was a brilliant idea, but the way he was talking he was suggesting that it was all his idea from the start, which it wasn't, we all designed the cooking event and we were going through with it, I think they were taking credit for our ideas in some cases, and he wasn't giving us a mention about starting it when he was saying this to the service users. Maybe it's just a small point, but I guess we will have to see if the story makes the chronicle, it would be nice if they could carry it on, only three people turned up today but if they enjoyed it as much as they said they did then they will tell their friends, and it can go on from there.

I still feel a bit cynical towards Voluntary. I get the impression they will hijack this idea and try and use it themselves, which is fine, it's a good idea, and we are working for Voluntary, I just would have liked maybe a thank you from the manager. He didn't seem overly interested in talking to us, but I did manage to get him to try a piece of banana cake, and he said he liked it.

See how things go, I guess. We finished up and had to clear everything up. I didn't do much tidying up, I think I was a bit drained from telling people to do things and monitoring the cooking. I wrote out the recipe for the banana cake for the service user, she was over the moon with it, we had tons of cake and chilli left over so we offered people a box of chilli to take home, she took a box, but no one else did.

My student colleagues said I could keep all the ingredients that were left over, which was very nice of them, and I had three boxes of chilli to take home so I was sorted for my tea! I was really happy today, I thought everyone worked really hard, and the efforts paid off, it had been a hard slog getting everything ready, but this had really been worth it, I felt we had achieved exactly what we had wanted to, educating and getting service users involved with healthy eating, and this wasn't rocket science, this was basic stuff, and extremely easy cooking, and this is what I wanted to get across to people, and I think it worked, all the service users said they would come again and had really enjoyed it, we must be doing something right!

I wish I could get involved in something like this again if it happens in the near future. I hope our efforts don't go to waste, it would be a good thing to keep running, I just think that with my other time commitments I wouldn't be able to devote any to helping out, but you never know, I have to wait and see. It will be interesting to see what story comes out in the chronicle, as the guy who took the picture didn't ask us any questions about what we were doing, so I guess Voluntary has filled them in as to what it's all about, watch this space I reckon!

I felt so good about today, that I was still awake at 1am, coincidentally, the time that an earthquake decided to erupt all over the country!

27/2

Other placement day, at least I got a parking space this time, the JCB's had all gone, and the pub had been knocked down so there was plenty of space to park. It felt strange walking in today, I guess cos I hadn't been here last week, I said hello to everyone and grabbed myself a cup of tea. There wasn't many people here today, I saw the chap who we had helped go and get some breakfast a few weeks ago, and who had felt ill, he seemed very pleased to see me, he had been in hospital and I was worried about him a few weeks ago, but here he was, and he was smiling away. I asked him how he was, he said he was fine, he was just in hospital for observations.

Had a quick chat to my student colleague, and decided we were going to go on another walk! I really enjoyed it a few weeks ago, and there were two people going from here, so we asked if we could join them, they said it was fine.

We met up at the same place again, but this walk was slightly different, just sort of the reverse of the last walk I went on, it was good to get some fresh air, and there were quite a few different people out on this walk this week, but most seemed to keep themselves to themselves, I wasn't comfortable with trying to chalk up a conversation with them so I mainly stuck with the two people from the placement and chatted to them.

When we got back, there wasn't much happening. I was speaking to the guy who seems obsessed with his home town and that everything is his fault, I tried to get him out of this way of thinking and tried to get him on other subjects, but he wasn't interested, I asked him why he was so interested in his home town, he said it was because his brother lived there. I felt a bit more comfortable with this guy now. I felt sorry for him as he was obviously locked in some kind of cycle of thoughts that he just couldn't seem to break out of, but in a way he seemed comfortable with this, he was harmless, but I wish I could get him onto other subjects.

I got round a few people today, didn't push myself on anyone, but just kind of chatted to people when they wanted to chat to me, it works a lot better this way, the group is very laid back, and a lot were asleep for most of the day, but I managed to talk to a good number of people.

One of the regular members of the group was back from the hospital, the one who had previously been running up to me and talking at me about all sorts, I couldn't understand her at the time, but she was back and said hello to me, she seemed quite medicated, and not her usual self, she was sat in the seat and looked quite tired, indeed she even nodded off a few times. I felt sorry for her, she was clearly medicated quite a bit, and it had taken its toll, but she had certainly quietened down since the last time I saw her!

The last order of the day was sorting out the day trips for where people wanted to go, that was a huge kerfuffle, and was done by individual votes, people putting their hands up in the air. I would like to be involved in one of the day trips, but I'm not sure I will still be there by the time one gets organised. It was finally decided that there would be five trips in the year, the most votes got put down, and the list was done.

An old chap came up to the organiser who was organising the voting and writing down the destinations. I knew from a few weeks ago that this guy really wanted to go to an aircraft and war museum, the museum had got hardly any votes, so it wasn't on the list, the organiser said he was sorry that it wasn't on the list, and the old chap said 'It's OK, I didn't even vote myself', he looked really miserable with himself, and I felt so sorry for him, it was clear that he was never going to go to the museum any other way, I almost felt like jumping up and saying 'I'll take you!' That really did make me think. But what could I do, it was a voting system, and unfortunately that's just the way it went.

The manager sat next to me and asked me how to spell one of the five destinations, he sort of whispered to me in a joking manner **'it doesn't really matter which destinations I write down, no one will remember what they voted for anyway!'** at the time I sort of laughed this comment off, but now I'm thinking about it, that was quite an inappropriate thing to say, yes I guess it was funny, but I'm not sure if he meant it seriously or not, or whether he was having a dig at some of the people.

I'm not sure in general how to take this guy, he does a lot for the people, but then there seems to be this other side to him that doesn't quite sit right, maybe its just me, but that sort of comment just kind of stuck in my head as I was driving home. I won't be returning to this place for another six weeks, I felt quite bad about this, I'm finding this is the hardest thing to accept as I get more used to the people, I feel I should be coming more often, but its just a time thing, I have to have time for myself so I try not to feel guilty about it.

When I returned back home, I noticed there was an email from my lecturer, requesting to see the three of us about the email we wrote.

Should be interesting; be interesting to have another lecturer's point of view on how we feel we have been treated at Voluntary!

28/2

<u>Uncle Pat</u>: **Most things in life, good and bad, just kinda' happen to ya'.**

(Cocktail, 1988)

Two events on today, the presentation at the workshop and I was going to meet my befriendee afterwards for a coffee!

I didn't feel nervous or anxious at all today, I thought the presentation would be much more relaxed and wasn't worried at all. I was too busy to be worried, I feel I have so much on my plate at the minute I just haven't got the time to devote to being anxious. I had a nightmare rushing into town, and had to park up at the multi storey car park, which I never usually do, but I had to as I was meeting my other colleagues for a quick chat before the presentation just to go over a few things. I hadn't prepared anything, I was just going to chat about things we had done, so I guess that took the edge of things a bit, and we were going to present in a canteen so there was going to be no projector or PowerPoint presentation. I had prepared a slide show on PowerPoint just to run in the background, so I had packed my laptop for that purpose.

Got to the coffee shop, and we just went over a few things, we were all quite happy about the presentation I think; I knew it was going to be a lot more relaxed.

We got to the place and introduced ourselves to a few of the workers, then went into the canteen. We didn't stand up, we thought it best to just sit at one of the central tables and make it seem quite informal. There was quite a good turnout to be fair, at least fifteen people, we just each said our bit really, it wasn't planned as such, we just kind of discussed our own experiences and some of the groups that were available, I mentioned about the cooking we had done and passed around some of the menus. I felt quite bad, as some of the workers said that they couldn't read very well and couldn't understand what the menu was about, so I tried to explain to them how our cooking idea could be something that could take off in the weeks to come.

It was difficult at times because more than one worker would be speaking, and it was difficult to understand what they were saying, but we tried to do the best we could. One lady didn't quite grasp about the groups, and kept asking us to write it down for her, even though we had handed out some leaflets showing her the times and days. She couldn't help it, and I could hear some groans from other people in the room each time she asked if we could write it down for her. I felt sorry for her, but we did write it down and she seemed very keen on coming. After the presentation a few other people came up to us and asked how they could be involved in some of the groups.

I think a lot of the people there wouldn't be able to go to Voluntary because of their work commitments, but there was definitely some interest, and we never expected everyone to suddenly stand up and all go marching down to Voluntary, but if we can just reach out to a few people, then I think that we have achieved what we set out to. The people there were very friendly, and I didn't feel nervous at all, a very friendly atmosphere, and a job well done, after we had left we decided to go for another coffee for a debriefing.

2:45pm

After I had left my colleagues, I had to go and meet my befriendee in the square. I turned up dead on time, and he turned up almost exactly afterwards. He wanted to go to Starbucks again, so in we went. I was still carrying my laptop with me in its bag, and as I paid for my tea I knocked over a huge pile of gift certificates. I tried to awkwardly pick them back up, and tried to put them back in order, but ended up just having to put them in a big mess of a pile on the counter and sheepishly walked over to where my befriendee was sat, not a good start to the afternoon!

Things went off to a great start again, he was hoping to be moving out of his flat soon into a newer flat closer to his workplace. He seemed very lively and talkative, and we managed to keep a good flow of conversation for a good amount of time, things were progressing well, and then we hit a brick wall again, things turned very silent. I decided to try and utilise this silence more today, and not rush into saying too much. At first it felt awkward.. then more awkward, then I found myself trying to prompt him again and ask him things, it was clear he wasn't going to say much any more, this was strange I thought, maybe he was hearing voices, he seemed to be a bit more paranoid and couldn't look me in the eye very well, although this was usually his normal behaviour and I assumed the eye contact was just the Aspergers that he had low levels of. He said he had to leave soon, he quickly finished his drink, stood up and left, without even waiting for me to leave with him! He rushed out the door and walked away very quickly.

I couldn't work out what had gone on, had I done something wrong? Or was it simply that he didn't feel comfortable with me after a certain amount of time? Even though it was our University week for the next few weeks I had explained to him that I was willing to meet him on a Wednesday morning at 10am, so I guess I will have to wait till then and see how he is, I can't think whether the meeting went well or not, I feel confused about it all, I'm not sure he is getting any benefit from the meetings.

Well that was it for today, an interesting day anyway. I felt good about the presentation, not so good about the meeting, but a weight has been lifted off my shoulders in terms of the work load for Voluntary, now we just have a drop in at the Sixth Form College, and a car boot sale! No probs!

29/2

Had a meeting today after our morning in the university. This time it was with two of the lecturers, and it was about Voluntary again. They just wanted to discuss the email I had sent and the issues raised by it. It was good to talk to two lecturers, and I felt very supported, they basically got me thinking that I should really be ending my befriending before it carried on any further. I was having these thoughts anyway as I was worried about feeling guilty about not seeing my befriendee and working in my holiday and University time. They assured me that I shouldn't feel guilty and that I was supposed to be there as a volunteer and not a student, and volunteers can only give what time they can; I shouldn't feel pressured into anything. I said I was more concerned with how my befriendee would feel. The lecturers raised a good point which I hadn't thought of before, they said if I continued to see him and I didn't really want to be there, or I was worrying about other University work, then he would subconsciously pick up on these signals that I was giving off, and in the long run that could be more detrimental or damaging to his mental state. This was a good point, and I didn't really want to be in a position where I was meeting up with him just for the sake of it, if I was in his position then I would want a volunteer who had the free time to spend with me and had nothing else major to worry about, so this made sense to me. The lecturers were very helpful, and they were not trying to tell us what to do but merely help us in what decisions we wanted to make. They were fully supportive of the fact that we had done so much work for Voluntary, and said that we had clearly done above the normal amount of work that a normal volunteer would be asked to do.

I felt good after the meeting. Initially I felt like it seemed like a bit of a moan and I shouldn't really be wasting the lecturers' time with it, but they were really understanding, and I felt that we were right to be discussing our issues with Voluntary with them, and I was glad that we had. By the end of the meeting I had decided that I was going to call off my befriending. I simply didn't need that added pressure on me, and I should also think about my own health as well as a service user's! All in all a very helpful day as it helped clear my head of a few issues.

3/3

I rang Voluntary and spoke to the woman in charge of befriending; it was time to get assertive! My student colleague encouraged me to ring and to get it out of the way. I have a terrible habit sometimes of trying to leave things till later or put them off for no particular reason. Be strong, I thought! I told the woman straight, I couldn't carry on with the befriending, I was sorry to say it, but I explained how uni was getting quite busy and I needed to be in the right place mentally with it all. She said could I not still meet him on Wednesday like I had arranged, I said I couldn't which was a white lie as it turns out I do have this Wednesday off, but I thought I don't want to get caught in this trap again, if I'm going to be assertive, then this means being assertive and sticking to my plan! No I said, I said I was still at University and I just couldn't do it, and then after that it was the Easter holidays and I wasn't working in my holidays. She tried again to sort of suggest if I could do it in a few weeks' time, but I said that basically we had a six week gap now, where it was uni weeks and Easter holidays in-between, so I wasn't going to be much good to my befriendee if I carried on meeting him after a six week gap. I also explained to her that I wasn't sure he was getting much out of my meetings anyway, it could be early days I guess, but I thought it relevant to explain it all to her and try to be as honest as possible.

She wanted to try and get us to have an exit meeting with my befriendee present. I said this wasn't appropriate as what use could a meeting do? She agreed to send me an exit form, which I could just fill in and send back. She seemed to have got the message. She also recommended that I ring my befriendee to tell him I couldn't meet him, she was also going to ring him and explain. Initially I felt awkward agreeing to this, but I figure it's the least I can do for him, and it's the right thing to do, I will just be honest with him and explain about my University commitments.

She asked how our presentation at the workshop had gone, and I said it had gone well. She asked if anyone was going to give feedback about it. **FEEDBACK!?** I kind of stuttered, 'Err, well, when were next in we can tell you about it, yeah'. I hadn't expected this, this was typical of Voluntary, find out we have done something and they're suddenly interested in what went on. I was still doing well with my assertiveness, even when she asked when we were due to come in again. I simply stated we were in uni for two weeks, then it was our annual leave, and all we had left to do was to go to the drop in at Sixth Form College and organise a car boot sale. She seemed pleased at that (I should hope so, I've just added up my hours, and I've done a lot more than I needed to!). I think I handled the call quite well, I had stuck to my guns, I didn't want to sound shirty with her, I just told it like it is. I just didn't want to do it any more, I wasn't going to feel guilty about it either.

Thankfully that's sorted now. I breathed a sigh of relief, I could get on with worrying about the next few weeks of uni in the skills lab!

4/3

Thought I would ring my befriendee today just as a courtesy to go over what would have been said already by Voluntary. I left it a good day and a half just to make sure Voluntary would have contacted him, I didn't feel comfortable ringing him up and explaining everything to him first hand, so I thought give it a good day and a half just to make sure Voluntary had contacted him. I felt a bit worried ringing him up as I started to feel guilty that I was essentially saying 'I don't want to work with you any more'. I know what the University lecturers said but it was still hard to get these thoughts out of my head. I had originally thought of not ringing him at all and just leaving Voluntary to sort it out, but my conscience got the better of me and I had to ring him, I don't think I could live with myself if I didn't ring him, it just didn't seem the right thing to do.

So I call him up, thinking it would be an easy enough call, just tell him I'm busy at University, and tell the truth. The call basically starts something like this:

ME: Hi it's Jack, I'm just seeing how you are and whether 'NAME of Voluntary worker' **(real name removed to protect the incompetent)** has contacted you.

BEFRIENDEE: Hi, no she hasn't.

Slightly dramatic pause......

Oh dear, my worst nightmare had come true, no one had contacted him! I felt incredibly awkward all of a sudden, I just had to carry on and be strong.

BEFRIENDEE: Are we still meeting tomorrow?

ME: Ah, well that's what the call was about really, I can't meet you any more, I'm just so busy with University at the minute, and I just can't devote any time to befriending I'm afraid.

BEFRIENDEE: Oh…

ME: And I don't think it's fair on you if I'm meeting up with you with all my University commitments at the back of my mind.

BEFRIENDEE: No, that's fair enough; if you have University commitments then you need to concentrate on them.

I thought he was taking the news quite well really.

ME: So no one has contacted you then?

BEFRIENDEE: No… When will I get another befriender?

ME: (stuttering a bit) I'm not sure, but 'worker at Voluntary'**(real name removed to protect the incompetent)** should be contacting you to try and arrange someone else for you. I'm really sorry but I just can't manage the time at the minute, but best of luck with everything and it was nice meeting you.

BEFRIENDEE: OK, that's OK, thanks again.

I hang up, god I felt really guilty! That poor bloke, he was going to turn up tomorrow. I was more annoyed at Voluntary, and no one had contacted him! Unbelievable! She had a whole day and a half to contact him! What the hell was going on! It was her responsibility to contact him too, what if I hadn't rung him, he would have turned up on his own in the square and felt let down when I didn't show. I thought this was very bad practice, I was so angry, but part of me just thought it was typical Voluntary, how unprofessional was that though!   I felt sorry for my befriendee, he was clearly being managed by a group of unprofessionals that couldn't be bothered to pick up the phone and tell him what had gone on.

Part of me thought that she was intentionally leaving it up to me to ring my befriendee, but then I thought, that really shouldn't be my job should it? If I am a volunteer working for Voluntary, then as she stated my call to my befriendee should really just be a courtesy call, just to say that I wouldn't be meeting up with him any more. I don't work for Voluntary, and I'm not paid to work for Voluntary, so it's not my responsibility to be ringing up my befriendee. God I was angry! I had a good mind to ring them up and ask why they hadn't called him, but I didn't, I thought there is no point, they're not going to change, I just was glad I was finishing my placement with them soon. I had done enough, I was tired of their incompetency, I was simply relieved to have cut my ties with my befriendee. That sounds bad, but as I keep telling myself I have done a lot for Voluntary, and I needed to focus myself back on my University work. I wasn't superman, I couldn't just do everything, I needed to focus on my University work and be grateful for the experiences I had gained, good and bad, from Voluntary at this present moment in time.

6/3

Woke up feeling a bit stressed, my student colleague texted me to say that we got in the paper today!!

Pretty pleased really, although I do have to say, as predicted Voluntary took all the credit for the event, saying that they organised it all! And we are classed as STAFF!! I thought we were supposed to be volunteers? They didn't even say we were students. I realise that we work for Voluntary in our current capacity, but at the end of the day we organised this whole thing, created the menus, organised people to come, organised buying the food, organised the venue, and then Voluntary swan in, organise the paper and say that they are looking to expand the scheme! They didn't even come up with the idea and now suddenly they are looking to expand it! Well I was a little disappointed, but still pleased that we got in the paper, it shows we achieved something and we at least got some recognition, even though we didn't get the credit for it. Oh well, what more can I expect from Voluntary, we are used simply as tools for their promotion. I guess that's the way it works sometimes, at least I know what we put into it.

10/4

It's been quite some time since my last diary entry, due to the nature of the course. I have had to be in University for a number of weeks, so technically we have not been on placement. I even managed to have a nice two week break over Easter!

The boot sale is looming, and today I am going round to one of my student colleagues to go and price up the remainder of the items. I have been collecting items for a number of weeks now, luckily a lot of the other students in my group have kindly donated lots of stuff, so we have more than enough for the boot sale which is due to be done this Sunday. I had received an email a few days ago from Voluntary saying that they had a reporter who was very interested in taking our picture for it! Another possibility of getting in the paper! That should be interesting.

I had priced up most of the stuff at my house, so this trip wasn't going to take too long. My colleague had also managed to get hold of an impressive amount of items. It didn't take us long to price everything, it was good to get out of the house actually, I had been staring at all this boot sale stuff for most of the day, and I thought I'd get a slight change of scenery, looking at yet more boot sale stuff but at least it would be in a different location! Once everything was priced up, it was just a question of waiting to see what the weather would be like for Sunday; the forecast was not good, showers! We were determined to go ahead and do it anyway, this was my second to last commitment for Voluntary and I really wanted to get it out of the way!

12/4

I packed the car up tonight, full of all the boot sale stuff. Our neighbour was getting dropped off by a friend in his car, the friend could see I was packing all this gear into the car and he started enquiring as to how much I wanted for the CD rack! I said three quid; he got out of his car to have a look at it! I thought this would be good, make a quick sale before the morning of the boot sale! Alas, it wasn't quite what he was after, the stand couldn't stand on its own, I think it was supposed to be screwed to the wall, damn it! I had a job squeezing it into my car! My student colleague texted me to say she had even more stuff to bring! I wasn't sure if I would fit it all in the car, as it was at absolute bursting point!

13/4

Day of the boot sale!

06:15am – What does the o stand for? OHHH my god it's early!!

Boot sales. I do love a good boot sale, I usually get around a lot when the weather's better, mainly for buying, but I have sold at boot sales more times than I care to remember, but this morning I felt like shit. Granted it probably didn't help that I had consumed three cans of lager the night before, but getting up at 6am seemed to give me quite a shock to the system. I felt drained, part of me didn't really want to go ahead with it, which is a bit selfish of me, I guess it was just because of how knackered I felt! My colleague texted me to say that she also felt like shit! It wasn't just me then. I grabbed a flask of green tea and set off to pick my colleague up. Our other colleague we think was ill as we hadn't heard from her, so it was just going to be the two of us; at least it wasn't just me on my own! I must have been in a bit of a daze as I almost forgot to turn into where my colleague lived, I was tearing up the road towards the Harry Hotspur pub where the boot sale was, and almost missed her turning. I swung the car very hard into the turning and all the boot sale stuff crashed into the side of my car with a big loud bang, I really must be more careful in the mornings! Nothing was damaged though thankfully! And I made it in one piece.

Once I had picked up my colleague we set off again, towards the pub, in which there was...

NO–ONE.

Oh dear, there was an empty car park! No stalls in sight! A nervous laughter erupted in the car. OK; I had definitely seen the ad in the paper! But it was OK, I had a backup plan, there was another pub not too far from here that was also holding a sale, the pub just down the road. It was a smaller venue, so I was hoping it wasn't too packed, but I sped down there quickly and luckily there was plenty of space. I parked up and opened the boot. My colleague hadn't sold at a boot sale before so I said the most important thing was to get the table out and start setting things up. People were crowding round us very quickly, and I was trying to get everything out quickly. I felt a bit flustered, it had been a while since I sold at a boot sale, and I had forgotten how quickly people can crowd round!

Things got set up pretty quickly and we were rocking and rolling! I had even bought a new money belt off eBay especially for the occasion, however, it bust within ten minutes and I managed to throw all the change on the floor because it had developed a MASSIVE hole! Well that was three quid well spent! I had to just use my pockets, which were a bit fiddly, but all I could do.

Once everything was set up I had a quick look round myself. I didn't find anything to flog on eBay though! We got the signs up for Voluntary, and stuck them on the table and car. It looked quite good! A lady tried to barter me down for a steamer to 2 quid! TWO QUID!! I had priced it up at 3 quid, which was ridiculously cheap anyway, I said to her 2.50 and **IT IS FOR CHARITY YOU KNOW**! She suddenly looked quite guilty and said 'Oh I'm really sorry about that I didn't realise, here have 3 pounds, sorry'. I got her a bag for the item and she continued to apologise. I don't do a good barter, but I was thinking that it is for charity, so I should probably use this tactic again if people try and barter too much!

Towards the end of the sale a partially sighted man came along and had a chat to us. He was very interested in what we had to sell, and he knew about Voluntary when we told him about it and why we were raising funds for them. We showed him a lot of items, and he wanted to touch and feel everything to get a better idea of what the item was. He told me that a lot of people had spoken to him at other boot sales and asked him why he was coming to boot sales when he 'couldn't see', I thought that was a terrible thing to say, I said that to him, why shouldn't someone who is partially sighted come out and enjoy himself on a Sunday morning? Why should he just sit at home?

He was extremely chatty and he must have been at our stall for a good half an hour. He also asked me if I had worked with anyone with Aspergers syndrome, which I had (coincidentally my befriendee), he said he had the more gifted end of it and could remember dates and facts easily. I think he appreciated the company, he wasn't with anyone else, it was just him. As the cars were packing up and ready to go he asked me if I would walk him to the door of the pub, as he was going to have lunch there at 12pm and he wanted to get out of the way of the cars and be safe. I said sure, I felt really sorry for him, he wasn't with anyone and he was going to dine on his own, he did this every week apparently, he was a really nice bloke and I felt privileged to walk him to the pub door. Again its such a simple thing, but it was clear that not everyone treated this guy as a human being, just because he couldn't see as well as most of us, it was clear that some people judged him immediately, but as I had the chance to get to know him, I could see that he was an extremely intelligent man and simply wanted to enjoy himself and get out on a brisk Sunday morning and have a pub lunch, so who could blame him! After I walked him to the pub entrance he thanked me, he asked me my name, and wished me all the best, that really cheered me up, and he had seemed pleased with all his purchases, he purchased three items from us!

We were still making a few sales. Some people were packing up but there were still a few people about, I had to refuse to sell a Simpson's clock for a pound simply because it was a group of horrible little kids! The clock was originally £3, and I said they could buy it for £1.50, even that was ridiculously cheap, but they kept pestering me to sell it for a pound, so I just thought sod it, you're not getting it for less than £1.50! I never did sell it in the end, but the important thing is, I stuck to my principles!

I bumped into quite a lot of people I knew from the EBay circuit. I know a lot of dealers (not drug dealers!), and quite a few were out in force today, I also bumped into a friend I used to work with a long time ago. She chatted to me, but I could tell something was wrong, again I don't know if it's because of my training but there was something behind her eyes that I could just tell wasn't right, to me she seemed medicated and a bit vacant, not the friend I used to know at all, normally she would be very outgoing and bubbly, sure it was a Sunday morning and people do have their up and down days, but I just knew there was something more to this. We couldn't really talk much as there was a lot of hustle and bustle going on, but it did worry me.

12 o'clock came very quickly indeed, and we were in full swing of packing. My colleague had the genius idea of dumping all the unsold stock at a charity shop in town! Perfect, I wouldn't have to cart it all back to my house! We got everything packed, and it was off to town. Literally about five minutes after we had packed up it had started to chuck it down with rain! Perfect timing. We had added up our money for the day, and managed to get 77 quid raised for Voluntary, pretty good going for about four hours work, and in my view quite a lot of tat stock!

We got to the charity shop in town. It had a lovely big porch so we could dump everything under cover, there was a sign saying they did not like stuff left for them in plastic bags, luckily all our stuff was all in cardboard boxes, so I guess technically that would be OK! Anyway, we just dumped it all and drove off pretty quickly! That was it, done, car empty, success!

One down, one more to go, what a relief! I felt tired today, but felt good. It had felt good to chat to some people at the boot sale, and I think my colleague enjoyed it, having never sold at a boot sale before, we had a good laugh together and raised a decent amount, and I had done my bit for charity!

No reporter had turned up. This didn't surprise me, Voluntary didn't seem the best at organisation. I wasn't really bothered, it would have been nice to get in the paper again, but I didn't feel too bothered that they hadn't turned up, at the end of the day we had put the effort in, and we know what we did and we had the proof.

15/4

'There are things that I'd like to say, but I'm never talking to you again'

(Foo Fighters)

Today marks a seminal day in the history of my voluntary placements; my actual final day for Voluntary! After this I can kick back and leave the complex mess of organisation chaos and at times downright rudeness and disinterest behind. The final task is to go and set up a stand for Voluntary at the Sixth Form College, which was set up a long time ago. I realise today that I'm over my allotted hours for this placement, so technically I don't actually need to be here, I wouldn't have bothered but it will form a sense of closure, and it seems a shame to let other people down when it was organised well in advance. It shouldn't take too long anyway, and it won't be that stressful, I mean it is just a drop in!

I picked up my student colleague, and we had to go and get the display boards from Voluntary first and some badges and pins to hopefully sell. We talked briefly to the people at Voluntary and told them all about our boot sale success, they seemed very pleased (well of course they would, they didn't lift a finger, and we promoted their brand and raised money for them by dragging our asses out of bed at 6.30am to stand around and sell 'tat' to people). The manager was there and as usual I think he almost tried to smile but obviously found it too difficult so it came across as a slight sneer, and then he went back to looking at his monitor as though we were just a figment of his imagination. We had only just raised 77 pounds, but hey surely that much is worth a smile and a thank you ? Obviously not. One of the support workers was there too and she asked us how things were going with our course, it was clear that she wasn't really interested, just small talk really, so we got the boards and quickly made our exit. Next stop, Sixth Form.

It had started to rain. Earlier today I was fooled into thinking it was going to be a lovely summer's day, the sky was actually blue, and the sun was out, I even contemplated at one point putting sunglasses on, but it was a good job I hadn't, because as usual it had started to tip it down and the clouds had gone a very dismal grey. I had to re work out how to get to Sixth Form because for some reason the whole of the town is in disarray because they are altering the whole one way system. This was not good, I actually had to stop and think how to get into the Sixth Form from a completely different way, I didn't need this hassle today. We finally got to the Sixth Form only to find that the main entrance to the car park now had a shiny blue sign cemented into the ground reading 'no entry'. Our other student colleague was waiting there, and we realised we couldn't actually drive in through the front. There was a street up ahead but that was also no entry. We looked puzzled at each other, we looked at our other student colleague waiting patiently outside the Sixth Form, almost as though we were willing her to help us with an answer on what we could do next! Almost like we were trying to evoke some telekinesis with us sat in the middle of the road just sort of urging her on for an answer.

There was no other option, I had to break the law! I quickly drove down the side street where it said no entry. There was no one there so it was safe, I just couldn't think how else to approach the Sixth Form at all! I quickly spun it round the right way and entered the Sixth Form car park through the side entrance, going past a sign that said permit holders only! Oh Dear! Luckily there was a car park attendant to speak to, we just explained we had no permit and needed to do a presentation, he was fine with that, and told us to sling the car in a nearby space, which I completely messed up so I had to squeeze out of my door almost holding in my breath as it was ridiculously close to the other car, oh well, at least we were here! Time to grab the stuff and head to reception!

We met up with the Sixth Form teacher and she said she thought it would be best to be placed not in the main hall as previously suggested but to go into the library the other side of the street in the newer area of the Sixth Form. Fair enough, we had to leg it across to the other side as it was absolutely chucking it down! We were given a fairly nice spot in the library, although it was right next to the entrance so every time the door opened it got pretty cold! I set up pretty quickly, and put the laptop on the table running a load of slides that I had prepared previously for the workshop presentation but hadn't actually used. And that was it, all ready to go, we all sat down and waited for some people to have a look and possibly a chat with us.

We waited…

And we waited…

Then we took lots of pictures...

And then we waited...

…………………………….

………………………………………………….

Then we took a few more pictures…

And then we waited…

We waited some more.

We thought about waiting, and then we did actually wait a bit more.

Almost an hour had passed, this was hopeless, absolutely no one had bothered or even looked, in fact the only comment we had was a passing comment from a lad who spotted a picture of monopoly on the laptop screen and had uttered 'err, monopoly'. Well that was great, we were fed up with this, we were just sat like lemons, we made the decision to start packing up. It was clear that no one was going to bother, so why should we waste our time even more ?

Towards the end when we were packing up the Sixth Form teacher came over and asked how it had gone, well, we had to be honest, she was very understanding but thanked us anyway, she even said she would write up something for us to say about what we had achieved, so we could use it as evidence for our portfolio, so that was one thing, we had to just chalk this one up to experience, at least we had done our bit, there was no point wasting any more time.

Next stop Voluntary, to tell them the good news! Had to go half way around town again because of the stupid new system in place. Got up to to the offices again, there was only the manager and another worker in the office, so we explained that it wasn't really much of a success but we had tried.

The manager as usual sort of looked at us as though he had seen us before, but again sort of brushed us off as another potential figment of his imagination and then went back to clicking his mouse and staring at the screen, pretending to do some work. I wonder if he actually knows our names. I wonder if he actually knows what we have done for Voluntary these last few months, I wonder if he realises how much we have worked our asses off organising things and getting the message out to people on his behalf. I seriously doubt he does, and I guess he will never realise, because I certainly won't be telling him. I've had enough, there's only so much someone can take without getting any sense of purpose. I'm not expecting him to jump up out of his seat and hug us all, but hey, the least we could expect is a smile and a thank you surely? We even gave him the leftover signs from the car boot sale that we had laminated up. He looked at these as though they were some strange kind of space age device. He looked quite disgruntled, I'm not actually sure if this man knows where he is. Maybe he's in his own lucid dream where he thinks that he can manipulate any object or person around him, and is having difficulty with it as he is trying to make us all disappear, and conjure up his true dream environment of him sitting on his own private island with his yacht and a pint of beer. Is this man the boss, or does he just think he is? Who cares anyway, this just said it all today, clearly he couldn't give a toss, I felt like just telling him to piss off, I really did, and I really don't get externally angry very often. I could have just stayed in bed today, and had my own fun in my OWN dream world!

I could have been doing a million things today, I could have actually done ANYTHING rather than waste my time messing about with a stand that no one was interested in, and people who actually worked for the company also weren't interested, so basically the whole thing was redundant. As we said our goodbyes (I'm not actually sure he said goodbye) by this point I thought he could shove it.

I walked down those stairs dejected and unwanted. I had put literally hours and hours into the presentation work, I had compiled the boot sale posters, the menus for the cooking event, two sets of power points, numerous other things, and got absolutely no thanks at all. As we walked downstairs there was a comments box for Voluntary where you could rate your experience, a red card being the worst. My student colleague put in about three or four red cards which just summed it up really! She agreed with me, she felt pretty dejected, I mean what was the point? Why had we gone to all this trouble, who were we helping? I was glad this was the last 'event'. I was ready to go home, I never wanted to see this building again now, I was totally fed up, I might as well have just watched paint dry for three hours and then told a blank wall my progress in watching the paint dry, that's what it felt like; utterly, utterly pointless.

I will continue to go to any talks that Voluntary put on, because that will help me in my ongoing development and education, but I certainly won't be telling people that Voluntary are a good company to work for. I don't see why I should, in this day and age aren't we supposed to be treating all people equal. Voluntary themselves even promote that they are non judgemental to people, but they certainly judged us, and we were certainly categorised and put in a neat little box labelled 'student labour', and that's just wrong. We needed to feel a part of the team, and we just weren't, its like we were in our own little world helping them out, not being involved with any service users or other volunteers.

Well I think that's enough, I'm too mad now, I need to go and chill out and watch a film or just clear my mind. At least I've got closure now, it hasn't ended the best, but I've certainly learnt a lot about myself and how people can treat you, so I will take that away with me, and try and focus myself on what I have achieved rather than what I haven't. At the end of the day I know I can work well on my own initiative, and I know that as a team we can get a lot of stuff done, but a lot of the time it has been quite a miserable and hard going placement, just from the sheer lack of support and alienation at times. I think it's time for a green tea.

This has calmed me down a bit. I think that's the last I can say about Voluntary, and it has been an adventure, just not a particularly pleasant one.

16/4

The other placement today, for the last time! This marks the last day of all my placement work, and I felt relieved as I was driving there today. Blasting out Abba on my radio, I actually felt glad, looking back it had been a long three months, and I had been involved in a whole manner of activities and organising. I felt like a break and a rest.

When I got there my student colleague had also just arrived. Upon entering the building it seemed quite busy, there were a few familiar faces, and the manager was there, he seemed pleased to see us. Before we had chance to get a cup of tea he came up to us and said he needed to speak to us, he needed to fill us in on what had happened over the past few weeks. He looked quite serious and stared at us from time to time with some strange awkward silences. At times it was like being in a strange film, it was almost as like he was pausing at crucial moments for his close up and then eventually telling us more of the plot, and it was a little surreal for such an early hour of the day. For some reason he had to keep addressing us by our first names, it wasn't like he didn't know who we were, but he still seemed to need to state our names almost at the end of every sentence.

We were ushered to the back room, and he began explaining how one of the members had been banned from the group entirely. As he was telling us this, he seemed to be pacing around and stopping randomly, almost as though he was trying to build up the anticipation of what he was about to say. There was another long silence. One of the guys I had spoken to in the early weeks had suffered two strokes. I felt quite sad, he was a nice chap, and seemed in good health when I last saw him. It was good to catch up on all the news though, no matter how strange the delivery, after that, it was time for a cuppa, and a chance to sit. And sit some more.

There was another chap that came up to me who I had helped take down for lunch all those weeks ago, he remembered me, and said he wanted to show me some recent purchases he had made. He ushered me to the far end of the building and I willingly followed.

For some INSANE reason I started to get a bit panicky as I was led to a room I hadn't actually properly been into, in fact, I wasn't sure what this room was for! For an absolute SPLIT second, I thought that he was going to lock me in this room and take a swing at me, I don't know why this thought suddenly smashed its way into my brain, I guess it's like the same idiotic thought processes that enter my brain when I'm 30,000 feet in the air and thinking the plane's engines are suddenly going to blow up. He was probably one of the kindest gentlemen I have ever met. I think at times my brain must have a meltdown; this was one of those times.

When I got to the room there was a huge pile of neat shirts in the corner from Next and River Island. He had purchased a good handful of shirts for hardly any monetary exchange, he was extremely pleased to tell me about his new found purchases and we quickly sifted through the jackets and shirts and discussed the current pricing structures of the key players in the clothing industry. We both agreed that he had truly experienced a fantastic bargain, and that he would certainly be kitted out for the summer months to come with a good range of new clothing at a bargain price. It was then time to grab a cup of tea.

9.45am and it was time to go for another walk with some of the members. This really does break up the day, and it's a good bit of exercise too. This week there didn't seem to be as many people walking, I guess the weather put them off a bit. A longer walk than usual, it took a good hour and a half off our day, and luckily it didn't rain.

On our way back we went through the car boot sale again, but no joy in finding any rare antiques. I did manage to grab a huge box of tomatoes for two quid, so that can't be bad, a good bit of exercise and a bargain all on my last day!

When we got back it was time to mingle I guess, although, there wasn't really much to do, a lot of the people had already gone to sleep! I chatted with a few other people, it seems to be that the best place to chat sometimes is in the kitchen as people are getting themselves a cup of tea. There were a lot of new faces today. I didn't impose upon their space, and just sort of left them to their own devices, they seemed quite content with what they were doing.

I felt like I had failed in the healthy living eating, I don't think there was any way that people were going to change round here, as I look at everyone tucking into cakes and drinking fizzy pop. It would appear that my University teaching is correct, you can't change people who are not ready or wanting to change, the chip shop was still the most popular choice for most people.

Towards the end of the day, the chap with his kid was there, and as usual she was getting fed all kinds of junk food and everyone was wondering why she wouldn't eat her proper lunch when it came round to it! He even asked his dad (who was sitting by him) if he could get him a can of pop, now this was strange because it was about four steps to go and get a can of pop, but he seemed to be unable to do this. Now I'm all for people doing favours for others, but this was certainly not going to empower him to take control of his own life if he couldn't get up himself and get himself a can, he said he needed to watch his child, I joked that he could walk backwards to get the pop thus keeping a check on his child throughout. The joke didn't seem to go down to well. I noticed that his child kept staring at me, for some unknown reason. I started to feel quite self conscious, I decided to stare back, my colleague joked that she was trying to 'melt me'. It was a well known fact that I wasn't very keen on kids. I decided to stop staring as the situation was getting far too weird for my liking.

Just after that another woman walked up near us and said to another lady who was sat down 'you are in my seat'. The lady who was sat down looked quite flustered, she immediately got up, apologised and had to walk halfway down the room to sit in another chair. I thought that was a bit harsh! There is supposed to be a rule in this place that there is no hogging of chairs or claiming one all to yourself. This ruling had clearly bypassed this lady, as she sat down in her chair proud that she had evicted someone from her premises.

There was a lot of sitting around today. I wasn't feeling that great, in fact I was feeling quite bored, there was simply not a lot to do. A few people were reading books, one guy was playing with his phone, other people were chatting amongst themselves, and a few people were asleep. I felt alone again, I only had my student colleague to talk to, and I felt a bit out of place at times talking to her, because I felt we weren't really supposed to be here to talk to each other. I'm glad of the company, but I felt at times that we should be talking to the actual service users, but that wasn't really possible! This wasn't the best days to end everything. I could carry on and visit again next week, but I was over my hours, and I simply didn't feel like it. I really wanted a rest I'd decided, this seemed a bit foolish of me as it was only my first day back here, but I didn't see what I was getting out of this placement, and I felt like a spare part. The people are very friendly here but I feel I should be in a more hands on role.

I looked at the clock; I was going in 20 minutes! My student colleague and I were now sat opposite the guy who was with his child. The manager had come to sit by me, the guy was holding his child and talking to us, he was talking about his diabetes and how his blood sugar levels were at 28! I'd never known anyone's blood sugar to be so high, there he was clutching a can of Pepsi too, he started to say how he wished he could get off his anti psychotic medicine, and how he thought people were watching him all the time, he laughed and joked about how he used to think that aliens had taken over and were going to whisk him away to Buckingham palace. The manager said that he could clearly think rationally and obviously had some insight into his illness, and that his current thoughts were being managed. It was apparent to me that this guy wanted to talk about his feelings and experiences, but here we were in this open environment with everyone sat around, and everyone would be able to hear this guy. I thought maybe this guy would be better speaking to someone in a quieter area, rather than tell all his problems outright for all to hear, wasn't this a shocking failure of confidentiality? I guess if he's happy to discuss these issues, then it is up to him. The manager was trying to encourage him that he was doing well under his medication but he clearly needed to address his diabetes and speak with his doctor about why his levels were so high. The manager turned to me just as he got up to leave and told me to 'say something'.

'SAY SOMETHING!'

Had I heard right? Say what exactly? I could offer more words of encouragement sure, but this guy was halfway across the room! What did he want me to say, start shouting questions at him and start talking to him, trying to help him with everyone else in earshot! If this guy had come to me and said can I have a talk with you somewhere more private I would have been fine, but he didn't, and I didn't go over to ask, which could be a negative thing on my behalf, but I thought that was a terrible thing for the manager to say to me, putting me on the spot like that, and it was a terribly unsuitable location to be discussing these deeply personal issues. It was time to go home, that comment pissed me off a bit. Before I could actually say anything, the guy got up to change his daughter's nappy, so it wasn't the best time to say something even if I could! Honestly, I just wanted to go, I felt flat in mood, I don't know if I got anything out of today except closure in my own mind. I was glad I had come just this once to sort of finalise things, but I certainly wasn't coming again. The manager said I was welcome any time and he refused to say goodbye to me because he said he 'knew I would be back' and I am 'welcome any time'. I might come back, I'm certainly not ruling it out, maybe things might be better in the future, but at least I know a few people here and know that I will be welcome, maybe I need to come back when I've progressed a bit more in my course, and compare the difference, if any, in what I observe, but for now I'm closing a book on the placement, and having a break from the voluntary sector. That's it for now, I've done my bit, and I can now have a bit of time to myself to reflect on my experiences.

Diary Conclusion 17/4

I just wrote that, and it looks a bit too formal for a diary, maybe it should be more like:

Final Entry! 17/4

Or just:

17/4 Last Diary Entry!

There, a bit less formal or final! I suppose diaries in a sense never truly end, our entire lives are essentially a living diary, but for the purposes of this diary I feel it a good idea to sort of sum up the long journey of adventure from the start of the year to here, the shower ridden April. I would love to say it has been an invigorating adventure, one that has been full of joy and purpose, but it clearly hasn't, however it has certainly made me think about myself a bit more and about others and how they interact with one another, either good or bad, and I feel I have also seen how organisations are run, badly in some cases! The time has gone quickly, and looking back, although the Voluntary placement came to a bit of a sticky end in certain cases, it has taught me a few good lessons, and probably made me think more about assertiveness, and seeing how organisations treat 'students' rather than volunteers. I hope if students go to Voluntary in the future they will be better treated or notified of how we were viewed, so that they can improve their placements by working more closely with the people involved.

My biggest regret is not having worked with many of the service users with Voluntary. I will certainly not burn my bridges with Voluntary, and continue to go to any talks they put on, indeed just the other day they sent me a letter stating that they would have a talk on psychological trauma, and even a bowling evening for the volunteers. I think it is important to still be in touch with them, maybe one day I may even be able to go back to Voluntary and actually work as a volunteer, but somehow I always think I will be viewed as a student, however I will be more assertive if an opportunity like that comes up again, but I fear it is quite doubtful given the time constraints with this course. I have to be responsible and that means devoting the bulk of my time to this course and getting it passed!

Although I think in general principle I wouldn't feel comfortable working for them again just from the very nature of their attitude towards us, maybe it would be different another time, maybe it could be done better, but am I actually bothered about trying? The way people treat you makes a huge impression on you and your confidence. I got a distinct lack of support from the people there and it has made me quite bitter in wanting to help them again, but who loses out? The service users. I don't know, it's just not a comfortable place to be involved with, and I think it might just be best to leave them alone and concentrate my efforts in areas where I can help people more positively and not be used for a cheap labour approach and a marketing arm of a large charity.

Working with my two other colleagues I feel has strengthened our working relationship both in placement and at University and we have worked together extremely well. I can't imagine what it would have been like if it was just myself working for Voluntary! At least we have all been in it together, and had a laugh with it all when things have got really down. We have learnt things about our own abilities and we have been able to organise quite a lot of stuff when I think about it and this will obviously be invaluable in our ever developing skill base, so for that I am thankful.

It is interesting to compare and contrast both placements. The other placement is almost completely different to Voluntary! Granted not a lot happens most of the time, but at least it was an excellent chance to actually speak to the people that used the service. I'm never quite sure if I really got a true rapport with people there, but I like to think I did, with at least a few people. I guess it's hard only going there one day a week, it's not a great deal of time really to truly get to know people, but in the sense of sounding a little clichéd, I'd like to hope I made at least a small difference to people whilst I was there. I know I'm always welcome to come back whenever I wish, but as usual it's the time constraints, which is a shame, plus in a sense we are not really true volunteers in the real sense of the word. I know we chose where to be placed, but real volunteers would be going to these areas completely off their own back, whereas in a way we have had a small push in the right direction from the University, it is part of our course, we HAVE to go to a voluntary placement for this particular term, so in a small way, it would never truly be a real volunteer's experience, that is why I think in the future it would be great if I could choose to go somewhere totally of my own accord, and then I would have a great comparison.

Someone once said to me that it is really difficult to clarify or explain to someone what a mental health nurse does, or what particular 'skills' they have. I guess it is hard sometimes, it's hard to explain that some days all you literally did was sit down with someone and have a chat and a cup of tea with them, but there's obviously more to it than that, and I think the skills you carry with you are like a toolbox, and you're always adding to them, it's the only toolbox I'll ever carry as I'm absolutely crap at DIY. I feel these skills insidiously massaging themselves into my psyche, and sometimes it just seems to flow naturally, I guess that's a part of how the learning system is set up and how we absorb information through lectures and practical on the job training.

Well I actually think that I'm going to shut up and close this diary up, whoever is reading this I really do hope it wasn't too boring, and hope that you got something out of reading it, it was certainly an interesting time being involved in these placements, for better or worse, and I feel it's certainly a learning curve, and I hope you can see just how much effort and time can go into some of the things we had to set up. Granted it wasn't ideally supposed to be like that, but hey, shit happens right? It has been an adventure writing the diary too, certain things can be clarified so much easier in the written form, and I guess I'm grateful to my brain for allowing me to get all my thoughts down in some form of semi logical structure, in a way it's been like one big therapeutic channel to use for my emotions.

I will leave you with one last film quote from Ferris Bueller's Day Off, a quote I think we should all think about once in a while. I am even going to put it on its own separate page, to ensure a more formal closure!   And to keep you salivating in wonderment and gently probe your curiosity...

Thank you for your time; it has been an adventure...

Jack Bennington

'Life moves pretty fast, if you don't stop to take a look around once in a while, it could pass you by………………….'

Diary of Anecdotes

The following few pages are 100% totally genuine. On the Dementia ward placement, they kept a small diary of comments about the food and what the patients thought of particular meals. The idea was originally to assess the quality of the products on offer and also to see if any changes were going to be needed in the range and choice on offer. These comments are what most of the nursing staff at the time recorded as the patients were asked about particular food items they were eating, and general comments said during mealtimes.

Patient made a comment on steak served at tea time: "terrible that is", steak was very tough and fatty.

Followed up above comment by saying it was a "bloody lump of shit that was" as his plate was cleared away.

Patient cried out "I don't fucking care" when offered lunch.

"I'm ready for the knackers yard"

"This is very civilized"

"I'm very worried, my mother said she would meet me here to go into town, where the hell is she?"

"Look what she's done, she's poured tea in rice pudding, she's a silly old thing isn't she?"

"This place is lovely and warm here."

"I'm not going anywhere. I'm booked up till Christmas."

"I'm not eating any more, I have never eaten three big meals a day."

"This is my friend, we came together."

"What time do the pubs open ? Are you the landlord?"

"I've wet my trousers, I can't believe it, don't tell him!"

"Its so quiet here, what time is it open or am I late?"

"can you cut this food for me, it's so tough"

"I want more toast, give me more food now!"

"I haven't been fed today, I'm so hungry, please help."

"This is a lovely spread, thank the woman who did it for me."

"This tastes like a bullock and a giant rose."

"mmm, no. This is awful."

"I'm not a patient here, I've only lost my glasses."

"Just let me out that door and I'll go over and out."

"I just want to go to bloody bed, I'll be up early in the morning and
I will be off."

"Please let me have a fag."

"It's far too cold in here, get me my blazer please."

"Oh come on, it's time to go, I'm not bloody stopping here all
afternoon."

"Is my father–in–law coming here? He said we'd go for a picnic."

"My sister's had a car crash. Will you let me go and see her now?"

"It's hot, so bloody hot."

"I used to work for the queen and she even let me sleep in her bed."

"Ooh it's so hot, I feel dizzy!"

"I'm only here for my arthritis."

"They're going to trim me up later, I hope I've picked the right day!"

"These are those silly 'lip laps' (referring to hip protector pants)"

"This tea's too strong, I can't have it like this!"

"It's so hot here, I can't get used to this heat."

"The food is shit here, not fit for a tramp!"

"He's a bloody tart, you need to keep away from him."

"Bloody men, all the same, hard in the morning, limp at night."

"I got no knickers on."

"Glamour boy, big belly."

"She's worse than the lot of 'em, you egg 'em on you do!"

"She thinks I've got the balls."

"Glamour granny."

"He'd rather go dumb than blind."

"What do you do with five beans? You hold two in one hand, and two in the other hand, then one up the jacksee!"

"Can you take me to the hospital ? I can't kill you."

"I'm counting on you to get the ticket for my room, last time I was here my daughter did all that." (patient talking about going to bed).

"This soup is a bit carrot heavy."

"I don't eat this rubbish."

"That Pakistani lady just pulled her knickers down and wee'd on the floor right in front of me, how awful."

"He is my husband you bitch, wish I had never harmed him."

"I can't eat breakfast, I have had a major operation."

"She doesn't wear knickers, she's a woman of the night."

"Nurse, can you look at my knees, they're burning up with all this medication."

"The dog's been on its own all day. I must get back to him, my husband's doing a late shift."

"There's so much for tea, I can't eat it all, I'll save my sandwich for tomorrow."

"I'll break your bloody legs if you come near me."

"It's such a long way to Dudley."

"Look here comes my baby."

"I want water, give me water."

"Come on, you have to feel sorry for an old man."

"Ah, get your knickers off and open your legs again."

"Toilet, toilet, quick, I can never bloody find it."

"Have you got any lemonade? Ah, beautiful."

"Before I die I want to be a virgin again."

"Am I a man or a woman?"

"Can I have that bread to feed the birds?"

"That bloody brother of mine has gone and left me in here."

Mental Health

"This is such a lovely place, you all work so hard."

"The food is lovely, that's why I like coming here."

"Do you shave your husband, well you need the practice."

"A squirrel comes into my bedroom every night."

"I am not eating dry sandwich."

"You're the nastiest little bitch I have ever met!"

Lightning Source UK Ltd.
Milton Keynes UK
UKOW04f2006260118
316920UK00001B/19/P